PRAISE FOR

The Best Things Parents Do

"Drawing on her own rich personal and professional experiences, Kohl describes the typical predicaments today's parents face and offers practical strategies for coping with them."

—Lilian G. Katz, Ph.D., Professor Emerita of Early Childhood Education, Co-Director of ERIC Clearinghouse on Elementary & Early Childhood Education at the University of Illinois

"At a time when everyone, layperson and professional alike, seems to have endless advice for parents and be more than willing to point out shortcomings, *The Best Things Parents Do* speaks with a decidedly different and refreshing voice. This holds up a mirror that reflects love, compassion, and courage. Kohl writes, 'What a privilege it is to be the person in a child's life who looks past his weaknesses to see the gifts that will become the gateways for new development.' This, in fact, is exactly what she does for parents in this book.

The Best Things Parents Do is a 'must read' for every parent who has ever felt incompetent, discouraged, or overwhelmed—in other words, a 'must read' for every parent!"

—Wendy L. Ritchey, Ph.D., licensed psychologist, private practice

"I am impressed with Susan Kohl's ability to put herself in the parent's place with sensitivity and compassion. The ways in which Kohl introduces knowledge and insights from many sources reveals creativity and a rich knowledge in psychology, developmental theory, humor, and problems associated with everyday living. As her former teacher, I cherished her. I am deeply touched to have the opportunity to honor her."

—Mary B. Lane, Ed.D., Professor Emeritus, San Francisco State University and author of *Our Schools: Frontline for the 21st Century, Education for Parenting, and Understanding Human Development*

The
BeSt
ThiNGs
PAReNTS
Do

Ideas & Insights
from Real-World Parents

SUSAN ISAACS KOHL Foreword by **M.J. RYAN**

CONARI PRESS

To Carol,

whose love has awakened my appreciation
for the best things parents do

—

First published in 2004 by Conari Press,
an imprint of Red Wheel/Weiser, LLC
York Beach, ME
With offices at:
368 Congress St.
Boston, MA 02210
www.redwheelweiser.com

Library of Congress Cataloging-in-Publication Data

Kohl, Susan Isaacs.
  The best things parents do : ideas & insights from real-world parents
/ Susan Isaacs Kohl.
      p. cm.
Includes bibliographical references.
  ISBN 1-57324-902-5
  1. Parenting. 2. Parent and child. I. Title.
HQ755.8.K64 2004
649'.1--dc22

                              2003021937

Typeset in ITC Century Book, Bureau Grotesque, and Clarendon
Printed in Canada
TCP
  11 10 09 08 07 06 05 04
    8   7   6   5   4   3   2

TABLE OF CONTENTS

FOREWORD

The first time I met Susie Kohl was over the phone. I had applied for my daughter Ana Li to attend the Meher Schools, a place around the corner from where we live that teaches grades preschool through five. At the time, Ana was two and a half, had very little language, and was not yet toilet trained. She had been abandoned at birth in China and was severely neglected. When we got her at age thirteen months, she weighed only thirteen pounds and could not roll over from front to back. Since the moment the orphanage workers put her into my arms, she had not been separated from me or my husband, Don.

Susie called because she was the head of the preschool. "Having read Ana's application," her soft voice said, "I think it would be best if I come and meet her at your house." So she arrived on my doorstep and proceeded to crouch down to talk to Ana. They played together for a while, and Susie returned the next day for more of the same. Then she suggested that we bring Ana to see the classroom she would be in when no one but Susie was there. We did that for a few evenings so Ana could get accustomed to the room and toys. Finally the big day arrived—Ana goes to preschool—and the only person who had tears in his eyes and separation anxiety was Daddy, who cried all the way home.

Ana stayed in that room with Miss Susie, as she calls her, for three years. Today, she is in first grade—a bright, confident, talented child with no signs of her early trauma. Since that first phone call, Susie has been my trusted confidante and parenting advisor. I know that my child is happy and secure and that I am a better parent due in great part to Susie's counsel and care.

Early on in our relationship, I asked what I could do to make the transition from home to school a smooth one. She said, "The best thing you can do is spend twenty minutes with Ana in the morning with no agenda. The rest of the day will go more smoothly." And lo and behold, she was right. Not only was getting Ana out the door pretty painless, but I counted those twenty minutes a day our most precious times. We'd lie in bed together, looking out the skylight and talking about whatever drifted into Ana's mind. After that, every time I was stuck or confused, I would seek Susie out. Each time, I found her suggestions wise and effective.

Now that you know my story, you will understand why I can't recommend *The Best Things Parents Do* highly enough. I am so glad this book has been published. Now everyone can have the benefit of Susie's wisdom and experience. Susie Kohl has been a mother, a teacher, a teacher of teachers, a preschool administrator, and a writer of parenting articles and books for many years. She knows what she is talking about.

And what she is talking about is so important! How to support the becoming of this tiny, vulnerable being that has been entrusted to our care. How to support ourselves as we go through this miraculous and challenging process while doing all the other things we must in our lives. And how to navigate the complexity of it all without beating ourselves up with guilt or regret.

Susie, like me, comes from what psychologists call an asset-focused approach. What that means is that she knows it is better to focus on what is right and good—in ourselves and our children—and strengthen that, rather than look at our flaws, weaknesses, or failures, which is a deficit focus. That's the beauty of this book. It helps us realize what we do well now so we can do more of it, rather than getting bogged down in all that we "should" or "ought" to do.

Recently I read two things that emphasized the difference between an asset and a deficit approach. The first one was an article that said parents today are more anxious about "doing it right" than any other time in history. The second was the opening line of Dr. Benjamin Spock's famous baby-care book: "Trust yourself, you know more than you think."

So consider *The Best Things Parents Do* an antidote to parental anxiety, a hand to hold so that you can trust yourself as a parent more and more. The greater health and happiness of your kids will be their own reward. And that, in turn, will be a gift to the world at large.

—**M.J. RYAN, AUTHOR OF** THE POWER OF PATIENCE **AND** ATTITUDES OF GRATITUDE

ACKNOWLEDGMENTS

My work on *The Best Things Parents Do* inspired plentiful discussion and collaboration within my family. I am indebted to my son Matt, my daughters Gabrielle and Mari, my mother Mary, and my daughter-in-law Lana for letting me tell tales about them. In addition, my heartfelt thanks to Matt, Gabrielle, Mari, my son-in-law Peter, and family friend Sharon Hatami for contributing precious hours of their time to proofreading and offering important feedback. My husband, Jeff, whom I consider the best step-dad and grandfather I know, helped in so many ways that no thanks would ever be enough. I see my beloved family's support as a reflection of the joy and privilege I experience every day just having them in my life.

I am equally grateful to friends who shared information, expertise, and stories, and parents who became friends through our collaboration, especially: Ellen Evans, my partner in exploring all that's "best" for children; Ira Deitrick; Caryl and Michael Marks; Karen Milligan; Monika Kochowiec; Adell DePersia; Diane Frolov and Andy Schneider; Ann Reed; Cecilia Soares; Dana Evans; Denise Brooks; Kathy Dadachanji; Karen Love; Eric and Terry Hummel; Amanda Wall; Lily Remer; Maggie O'Hern; Aida Faria; Carolyn Newbergh and Kevin Fagan; Rosemary Kirbach; Margo McKenna; Sarah Truebridge; Carol Palley; Robineve Cole; Loel and Rob Miller; Lynn Tidd; Lisa Andrews; Tamara Freda; Steve Harrell; and Susie Smart. Thank you also to all those who are mentioned in this book and to those who gave me great scenarios that will have to appear in a sequel.

I want to thank my friend and fellow author, Jim Peterson, for introducing me to my wonderful new agent, Barbara Deal, and dear Mary Jane Ryan, for believing so wholeheartedly in the project, writing the foreword, and for introducing me to the wonderful, encouraging editors Jan Johnson and Jill Rogers.

Finally, my gratitude and love go to all the parents I engage with every day and those I've worked with throughout the years for working so hard to illuminate the path for parents now and in the future.

INTRODUCTION

You're a Better Parent Than You Think You Are

> Suspend whatever interest you may have in weakness and instead explore the intricate detail of your strengths.
>
> **MARCUS BUCKINGHAM AND DONALD CLIFTON**

You've heard of bird watchers and people watchers. Well, I'm a parent watcher. For more than thirty years, as a parent educator and consultant, I've observed the wonderful ways that parents find to love their children and support their growth. I want parents everywhere to see what I see. That's what *The Best Things Parents Do* is about: helping you and others who care for children to be aware of the great things you do. The book highlights the way that ordinary people develop extraordinary abilities as they meet the challenges of parenting at all stages of development.

The parents I watch would probably be surprised to find out how remarkable they truly are. When parents come to me about dilemmas with a child, they are often in a state of confusion and self-doubt. Parents today are bombarded by conflicting opinions from others, many of them experts. Is it any wonder they become anxious? In our culture, confusion is usually seen as a weakness, but I view taking time to think through a situation as a strength. Their confusion is a "first step" and a healthy response.

When parents think through confusion, they stretch themselves to learn. The parents I work with are often much better parents than they think they are. My job, as I see it, is to help them be aware of their strengths and encourage them in their reach for new growth. That's what I want this book to do for you as well.

The Best Things Parents Do is also intended as a love letter and a thank-you note to parents. It says, "These are the wonderful things I see that you do, even if you can't see them for yourself."

The premise that people need positive feedback and awareness of their strengths is understood today in almost every field of endeavor. Companies routinely give employees rewards for high performance, and many help people to diagnose their natural talents and expand upon their skills. In other areas of life, people who want to lose weight or exercise more are taught to applaud themselves for their efforts and note their tiniest new accomplishment. We have become experts in cheering ourselves on in almost every arena of life but child-rearing.

My Story Is Every Parent's Story

For most of us, trying to be the ideal parents is a humbling experience. It certainly was for me. When my children were young, my friends and I believed that we were doing things differently than our own parents had, creating perfect supportive environments. I was a zealot about the importance of "the family." From the time my children were small, I referred to our nuclear family as a magic circle. But the road took unexpected turns, and my marriage unraveled. I realized in anguish that I couldn't protect my children in magical ways, nor were their lives going to play out in the perfect ways I had imagined.

I was confused. I didn't know how to be a single parent and had serious doubts about whether I was up to the challenge. The phrase itself, "single parent," seemed an oxymoron to me. I had inherited the belief from my own family that parenting was something two people did together. But since I had to try to be a "whole parent unto myself," I tried to live one hour at a time. If I had allowed myself to wallow in the self-doubt I felt, I wouldn't have been able to encourage my children in their own growth. As a consequence, I was forced to look at my own strengths and note my successes. It turns out that encouraging is one of the things I've done best, with myself and others.

I am also resourceful. I began to look for support from other people who cared about my children. That's when my definitions of the words "parents" and "family" began to change. I discovered that lots of people were parenting my children, even if they hadn't earned the title through biology. Each of my kids took sustenance and love from significant people who were involved in their lives. I began to see that I wasn't alone and that those of us who care about children are related as family. And I've been on both sides. Over the years, I've parented countless youngsters. That's why, when this book refers to parents, it is really addressed to all people who have a caring relationship with a child.

In a sense, my story is every parent's story. We all begin with our own fantasy of what parenting will be like and what we want our children to be. Then, real life repeatedly dissolves the fantasy, and we arrive at new insights, form new attitudes, and try doing things differently. It's not always easy, but giving up our naïve beliefs offers us the privilege of knowing more. Obstacles, puzzles, and crises provide us the opportunity to more fully understand the wonder of human growth—our own and our children's—the way it actually is.

The Best Things Parents Do gives you the chance to change your whole perspective on parenting and to see yourself and the parents around you in a new light. Every time you read a chapter, you will have a chance to meditate on how the "best thing" described relates to you and the situations in your life. Take a little time for personal reflection by considering the questions and suggestions at the end of each section. These "reflections" link the material in the chapters to your experience as a parent and as a child. Taking the time to tune in to our childhood perceptions, even when painful, allows us to understand our automatic reactions better and see our children more clearly.

The book is divided into four parts. We begin by exploring the attitudes that help parents feel happy and become more sensitive in their roles. The second part looks at the positive ways parents relate to their children: things they actually do. The third part points out crucial ways parents need to care for themselves: the best things parents do to replenish themselves and nurture their own growth. Part four focuses on parents' abilities to support each other, work together, and help children contribute their gifts to the world.

This is not a book to gobble up and put aside. Read a chapter and think about how it relates to your life. How does it connect with the ways that you were treated as a child? What does it tell you about a child that you love as a parent, as a grandparent, or as a friend? What does it spur you to learn?

I Hope You Become a Parent Watcher

I imagine you looking around at the people you know (and don't know) and appreciating the ways that people relate well to children. If we all take note of the positive examples around us, our world will change. People will become more aware of how parents stretch themselves to understand children's needs and meet them. Starting to notice and share our perceptions of positive growth will spawn a new appreciation of parents and caregivers. Respect for parents, teachers, and caregivers will increase, and society will place a higher priority on meeting their needs. I see our appreciation of people who care for children going out as a huge wave of support that will change the ways we view ourselves. It starts with us, but I firmly believe that the positive parenting revolution is just beginning.

PART I

THe
BeST
ATTiTuDEs
PAReNTS
HoLD

The first step on our journey is examining our attitudes—the ones we have inherited from our families and our society—and the unique expectations that we bring to parenthood. We often choose to become parents because of the popular fantasy that having a child will complete us and nourish us with a special kind of love. Parenting is indeed a course in loving, but in order to grasp its lessons we have to be willing to adopt realistic and flexible attitudes.

Our society leads us to believe that if we buy the right books and child paraphernalia, parenting will be easy. Some parts of having a child may feel instantly rewarding. But when we discover that knowing what to do as a mother or father is actually one of the most difficult challenges we will ever face, some days are bound to be confusing. "Is something the matter with me?" "Is there something wrong with my child?" "Maybe my child doesn't love me." "If I make mistakes, will I damage her?" Realizing that these doubts are based on the naïve perspectives that our society promotes can help us support ourselves and learn more about human development.

Our attitudes underlie everything we do, so it is up to us to notice and transform them. One of the best things we can do is learn to examine and update our attitudes, but always in a compassionate way. The world may find fault with parents, but learning doesn't come from criticizing ourselves or our children. We aren't good parents because we bring all the right qualities to the job or because we learned from the perfect parents. We become better parents by embracing change and aiming for wisdom, not by avoiding mistakes. Part of the real excitement and fulfillment of parenting comes from observing growth—not just in our child, but in ourselves. As William James said, "The greatest discovery of any generation is that a human being can alter his life by altering his attitude."

CHAPTER 1

Progress, Not Perfection

Progress, Not Perfection

No one is going to grade you as a parent. No one is
keeping score. You don't have to do it perfectly. You will
make mistakes . . . Accept this truth and you will find
being a good parent much easier.

JOHN AND LINDA FRIEL

When I give a discipline workshop, new participants always arrive
looking a little nervous. I have learned to expect this. Talking about
how we handle our kids can make many of us feel self-critical. Who
would claim they do it well? And who among us doesn't make mistakes? Throughout these workshops, people sigh with audible relief
when they realize that other parents share the same frustrations they
do. No one gets it right all the time. Recognizing that the point is to
gain insight, not have instant answers, overrides the voice that tells
these parents that they aren't doing a good enough job.

It's rare to find anyone who doesn't have an inner critic poking
holes in her confidence as a parent. Why?

We receive virtually no feedback on what we are doing well.

- "Experts" set impossible standards that may have little to do
  with our everyday challenges.
- Psychologists often blame parents for children's emotional
  problems, offering no feedback on what mothers and fathers
  do well.
- Most frequently, we criticize ourselves because our parents
  criticized us. The more our parents found fault with what we

did, the louder and more insistently we will resist feeling good about ourselves as parents.

I am convinced that the first step in parental growth is becoming aware that the voice of the critic is not reality. Moreover, we can easily counter it. The problem is that most of us try to dismiss critical thoughts by pushing them aside. Denying critical thoughts can actually strengthen them. Instead, I have often recorded what my inner critic says so I can analyze the statements objectively.

If I listed my inner critic's views of my parenting right now (even though my children are grown), it might say:

- You're always saying the wrong thing to the kids.
- You trouble your kids by worrying about them.
- You should know the best ways to support them, but you don't.

The list could go on and on. When I look at my entries, I can easily see that the critic overstates its case by using words like "always" or "never" or "should." The goal of my critic is to make me believe that a good parent has to be all-knowing and perform perfectly. I can counter these absolutisms by remembering that:

- I don't always say the wrong thing.
- I try not to talk to my kids about my worries.
- I always try to listen and support my children, but some-
  times I make mistakes. I'm only human.

Examining our critical thoughts objectively defuses their power and allows us to start seeing ourselves in a kinder light. Criticizing ourselves or comparing ourselves or our children with others leads to confusion. One of the best things we can do is to adopt the attitude that parenting is a learning process, and that no one has the "right answers." Learning requires increasing our awareness and self-acceptance. In the meantime, we need to encourage ourselves the way we would a friend. A parent told me recently, "I always do my best as a parent when I feel relaxed and happy about myself."

Without judgment, notice the times when you question your parenting. Do you seek answers to your concerns, or simply make yourself feel bad?

To identify your critic and diminish its power, give a name to the inner voice that undermines your confidence. Saying "Thank you, Miss Perfection" or "Sure, Mr. Nitpicker" can aid you in recognizing your critical voice and combating it. Write a thank-you letter to yourself for all that you do.

Comparisons Confuse

> We hear about the birth of a child and ask questions
> like, "What did she have?" "How much did it weigh?"
> and "Did it have any hair?" The Athabaskan Indian hear
> of a birth and ask, "Who came?" From the beginning,
> there is a respect for the newborn as a full person.
>
> LISA DELPIT

When my son Matt was four or five months old, a friend and I used to get our infants together to "play." We would lay them facing each other on a blanket and watch what they did. Her daughter, Angel, was a few days younger than Matt but a little more physically advanced. She could creep forward to grab Matt's face or try to poke his eye while my friend and I discussed the latest things our babies were doing.

I discovered early that the most popular subject when new mothers gather tends to be babies' new accomplishments. Our cultural ideal that faster is better reaches its high point of absurdity with our expectations for our kids. Did it matter that Angel could poke Matt's eye before he could scoot to pull her ear? Watching several generations of children grow has proved to me that comparisons usually mean nothing. But they CAN confuse. What if I had formed the crazy idea at that point that Matt wasn't physically adept? Would I have tried to influence him later not to play soccer or climb Mt. Shasta with his dad? Thankfully, I ascribed no meaning to Angel's precocious scooting, and I'm sure it means little in her life now. I wish we could just watch our beautiful babies with reverence, wondering what uniqueness they have brought to the world.

Now that my children are adults, it's easier to see that the ways in which they varied in development had little to do with the people they became. But when they were young, I wondered how they could be so different. The illusion is that comparing will lead to important insights. But differentiating our kids more often has limiting and even negative effects.

The problem with comparisons is that they inevitably leave someone feeling labeled. The most intense comparisons our culture makes relate to children's intelligence. What parent doesn't want to think of his child as smart and able to compete for high grades? Success in school, however, doesn't necessarily reflect high or low intelligence. In her revolutionary book *How Your Child Is Smart*, Dr. Dawna Markova describes the varied learning patterns that children exhibit. Unfortunately, the schools are designed to meet the needs of visual or auditory learners, so those children are usually considered smarter. Markova recommends making provisions for learners who benefit from hands-on experience and have the need to move around. Understanding learning styles can prevent us from labeling children as less capable.

In the home, children often get cast in roles: one will be a good eater, while the other picks at her food; one loves to read, but the other isn't interested; one is outspoken, the other quiet and internal. Many of these roles are the result of well-meaning praise. "Look what a great eater he is!" It might be more helpful to note, "You seem hungry today." When a child observes that one role is taken, he will look for another way to find his identity. His natural tendencies may have been to eat or read ravenously, but observing that his sister is considered the "good" reader or eater can propel him in a different direction.

In his bestselling book *The Tipping Point*, Malcolm Gladwell points out that human beings are so complex we can't hold all their qualities in our minds. People behave differently in varying contexts and relationships, and many of their traits are contradictory. Who could take them all in? He says that the human mind has a kind of "reducing valve" that helps us simplify and solidify our image of a person, even though that person is constantly changing.

If we want to rise above our reducing valve, we can try not to confine our children to a particular image ("Johnny's very shy." "Tillie isn't organized."). Believing that comparisons between children are especially odious is one of the best attitudes we can hold. Think of each of them as a wellspring of fine qualities waiting to emerge. To stay mindful of their vast potentials, we can think of Ralph Waldo Emerson's quote: "What lies behind us and what lies before us are tiny matters compared to what lies within us." Our children are worthy of the same respect and tolerance we would offer to a friend.

Think back to your childhood. Did an adult ever attribute a negative quality to you? Were you able to overcome it?

I Wouldn't Talk
That Way to a Friend

**Speak when you are angry and you will make the best
speech you will ever regret.**

AMBROSE BIERCE

Cora considers herself efficient and fast-moving. Two of her daughters seem to take after her, but she thinks of her middle daughter, Phoebe, as dreamy and slow. "When the family's ready to leave on an outing, Phoebe may still be getting dressed," Cora says. "It can take an hour for her to make a sandwich for her lunch because she keeps talking to everyone. I worry about her because it seems like a twelve year old should be able to work faster. She's only in junior high now, but will it be safe for her to drive as a teenager? She may drive off the road into a tree." Phoebe's slowness sometimes makes Cora angry, and she's had to learn to control her temper. When she feels her frustration rising, she excuses herself and asks for a time-out.

"I know if I speak while I'm in a rage, I will say something that I'll regret, and it'll be too late to take it back. When I go in Phoebe's room an hour after she was supposed to clean it and there are still things all over the floor, I feel like saying, 'What's wrong with you? Are you blind, girl? You're so slow. Your sisters were finished a half hour ago.' But I try never to do that. It's okay to get angry, but it's not all right to make judgments about my daughter and shoot holes in her sense of self. I would never say those things to a friend, and I want to be just as respectful to my child."

I have seen Cora in one of her white rages and been amazed at her ability not to say a word. Later she can talk about what triggered her upset, but after she pauses, it doesn't come out as the other person's problem. She might tell Phoebe that she's frustrated because she hoped she would be ready on time. But she's learned only to do that after her upset has dissipated.

Sometimes when she's upset about Phoebe, Cora calls her "wisest friend" and asks for an "attitude adjustment." Her friend reminds her that Phoebe's a normal twelve year old, and it's okay for her to be different from Cora. She may take her time, but she's a good student and keeps up her responsibilities. She's generous and gets along with other people famously. After hearing her friend's perspective, Cora realizes she's been overreacting. She loves Phoebe, and she tries to keep in mind that her own need for speed is her problem. Cora doesn't want to cast her daughter in the role of the distractible family member. So she consciously tries to adopt a new attitude.

Getting angry about things our children do is inevitable. But discovering what triggers us and being careful not to insult or attack our children are among the best things we can do. Although as a parent Cora's responsibility is to guide Phoebe, she knows that criticizing in anger will only leave her daughter feeling discouraged and disrespected. If we pointed out our friends' flaws, we wouldn't have many close relationships. I like Phoebe's mental test of appropriateness: "Would I talk that way to a friend?" Just think of the things parents have traditionally said to children ("I can't believe you did that! What could you have been thinking? How could you be so stupid?") and how hostile and demeaning they would sound if one adult said them to another. (Unfortunately, some do.)

The old saying, "Think before you speak," expresses one of the most important attitudes we can hold. Words can sting as sharply as blows, and verbal abuse can have long-lasting effects. It's our responsibility as parents to build confidence, not destroy it, regardless of the provocation.

Keeping this in mind makes some people determine never to get angry at their children again. But dismissing anger from our emotional repertoire sets us up for a fall. Parenting is one of the most difficult tasks we can undertake, and its demands will provoke our anger sometimes. However, adopting the attitude that we need to understand what triggers anger, in order to learn to handle it appropriately, is one of the best things we can do. Becoming aware of the situations that set us off can even give us the ability to maintain more tolerance in stressful situations.

Learning to control our tongues is the foundation for preserving our relationships with our children and reinforcing their positive feelings toward themselves. Apologizing when we lose our tempers helps our children to understand that managing intense feelings takes work, and that everyone makes mistakes.

Take the time to record yourself a few times when you're asking your child to change her behavior. Hearing what you really sound like will make you more effective.

Everyone Makes Mistakes

**The man who makes no mistakes does not
usually make anything.**

THEODORE ROOSEVELT

On fourteen-year-old Meredith's championship basketball team, mistakes attract intense criticism. Her team represents the whole San Francisco Bay Area, and every year they qualify for the national tournament. At this level of competition, there is constant scrutiny of every play the girls make. Videotapes are shot of each game, mistakes are analyzed, and the girls are coached to improve their skills. Sometimes, parents even punish their daughters for making an error. Pressure! Pressure! Pressure!

How does Meredith's mother, Dawn, handle the times when everyone is yelling because her daughter's mistake cost the team a point? She tells Meredith not to worry, that everyone misses a basket sometimes—and the idea is to enjoy the game. "You want to know the truth, I don't care who wins," Dawn says. "I'm not involved to make her the star. Other people quit because they want their child to be the one who excels and gets the most time on the court. All they care about is their kid and how well they are doing. One parent got so mad at the referee he even brought a gun to a game. It's scary!" Dawn continues vehemently. "I only support Meredith playing basketball because she wants to. I care about all the girls and how they are feeling about their playing. It's an extraordinary commitment that they give, and it has to feel good to them."

Every year Dawn and her husband John ask Meredith if she wants to continue. Even though she could eventually win a college scholarship, they place no pressure on her to better her performance or even to stick with basketball. Interestingly, their reassuring attitudes toward mistakes have given Meredith a relaxed attitude during tight situations in the game, allowing her to exercise good judgment. "They've made her the team captain because people have noticed she can remain calm during hard plays," Dawn says. "When you know you're going to be yelled at for making a mistake, you get tense and you don't think clearly." Dawn and John both feel that mess-ups are an important part of the learning, and they've always told Meredith that.

In light of these attitudes, it's also interesting that Meredith is the only player who has stuck with the team since second grade. She is now considered the most valuable player. But being the best is still not the point for her parents. "If she quits tomorrow, there would be so much about people she has learned. In the beginning her team was all white, and now there are two white members. Last summer, the other girls gave her an honorary African-American name. Having been voted the team captain, she's had to learn a lot about leadership and being fair to people. She cares deeply about all the girls and how they are doing." So within this outrageously competitive atmosphere, Dawn and John have been able to instill their values of compassion, cooperation, and taking mistakes lightly in their daughter.

What is our attitude toward mistakes? Do we show a toddler how to wipe up the milk he spilt or regard him as someone trying to make our day miserable? The first time a child colors on a table do we teach her how to keep the marks on paper or get angry at her for misbehaving? Do we treat spelling errors as opportunities for learning?

Pressuring children not to make mistakes actually inhibits them from trying. The famous educator John Holt wrote a bestselling book called *How Children Fail*, chronicling how children give up on math problems because they have learned to be afraid of making an error. Students who are good at math learn that a mistake means you have to try something different and go on with confidence. That principle doesn't apply just to math, but to all of life. Believing that mistakes promote learning is one of the best attitudes we can hold for our children and ourselves. It helps us maintain confidence that our efforts count, no matter how many times we fail. As Theodore Roosevelt says in the quotation opening this chapter, people who don't make mistakes usually "don't make anything."

Picture a time when someone reacted with compassion to a mistake you regretted. What were your feelings? Note the times you feel patient with a child's errors and the times they frustrate you. How can you remind yourself of the value of mistakes?

Effort Counts

Schools should teach kids how to learn, and parents should teach them how to work by establishing work rules and a work ethic at home.

DR. MEL LEVINE

Corrine laughs when she talks about trying to get her son to take a break from homework. "I guess it's not the usual challenge, but Ahmed likes to work hard at his homework, and we have to remind him to take a rest between assignments." That's the role that Corrine and her husband Al have always taken in relation to their son's schoolwork. They have coached Ahmed on how to put in his best efforts by approaching assignments in an organized way and taking time for refreshment. They have also established routines: Homework gets done right away and takes precedence over sports or any extracurricular activities.

When Ahmed started junior high, Corrine asked him if she could help him keep track of assignments. She even worked with him on a filing system to store graded homework in sequence. Several times that system allowed Ahmed to correct his grade when a teacher had recorded his homework marks wrong. Ahmed learned he had the power to raise his grade by noticing his teacher's errors and showing her or him the actual assignment.

Ahmed's parents have always praised him for working hard on his homework and taking satisfaction from a job well done, rather than for being smart and doing things with ease. "We don't talk in terms of intelligence but how much Ahmed learns from doing his best, and how we enjoy the incredible things he comes up with in his assignments."

Their emphasis on effort reflects what research has found. Dr. Claudia M. Mueller and Dr. Carol S. Dweck, psychologists at Columbia University, warn that labeling children as "smart" propels them to keep trying to maintain the label. The psychologists' six 1998 studies of fifth graders showed that when children who have been labeled "intelligent" have a setback, they assume that they actually don't have the ability to meet the challenge. The studies conclude that praising hard work encourages children to believe they can do well in the long term.

Holding the attitude that effort counts and supporting our children in their work are among the best things that parents do. But it can be tricky. Assessing our own school experiences and becoming a good work consultant take insight and effort. My parents encouraged me by telling me how smart I was and how easily I could do anything. When I got to geometry and other tough subjects, I didn't realize that these subjects just called for greater effort, and I ended up with a C.

When I became a parent, I, too, told my children how smart they were. When they became adults, we discussed how being labeled "smart" can make children feel pressured. Luckily, I praised them for effort as well, and they remain hard workers today.

It's up to us to analyze our feelings about schoolwork and to decide whether our interventions will help or hurt. If we care more about grades than learning, we are apt to pressure our child, making him dislike schoolwork and put off homework. If we get frustrated and critical, we shouldn't be the one to help. On the other hand, if we take a laissez-faire approach, leaving her to figure out how to do her homework on her own, she can easily flounder. If helping our child with homework becomes stressful, the burden doesn't have to fall on us. This is especially true if our child experiences challenges with school work. Qualified learning centers and tutors should be able to diagnose the exact help a child needs.

In his book *A Mind at a Time,* learning expert Dr. Mel Levine talks about the many different ways that children need help with their schoolwork. A child who seems lazy often has problems generating and sustaining her mental output. Instead of being told to try harder, she needs encouragement and practical suggestions for controlling her mental energy. The basis of helping children lies in our attitude; we need to sympathetically understand that every mind learns differently and tune into their individual strengths and challenges. That way you can discover concrete ways to support them.

Think back to some of the skills you've had to struggle to learn. What motivated you to keep trying? How did a parent or another adult help you with learning challenges?

Chapter 2

Opt for Optimism

One Hour at a Time

> . . . Just for today I will be happy. I will not dwell on
> thoughts that depress me. . . .
>
> **EXCERPT FROM ORIGINAL ALANON CREDO**

Dining out one day with two toddlers and their parents, my husband
and I noticed a dramatic change in the parents' attitude as the meal
proceeded. After about a half hour of their sixteen month old crying
and standing up in her high chair, and their two year old demanding to
go outside, both mom and dad wore looks of defeat. They had looked
forward to going out to dinner, but now they blamed themselves for
their toddlers' behavior. They predicted that they would probably
never have a pleasant meal out of the house for years to come.

I am intimately familiar with this kind of thinking—it's called "con-
cretizing the projections of a negative experience out into time." A day
when my children argued incessantly was enough to convince me that
the rest of my life would be spent mediating disputes. If my daughter's
ear infection came back, I predicted that I would be trotting to the
doctor all winter and blamed myself for the recurring infections.

Concretization is created by pessimism, the tendency to see the
glass as half empty, rather than half full. Pessimism rises when we feel
powerless to manage a situation that spins out of control. Soon we're
in a fantasyland of unceasing hardship. The solution? An optimistic
attitude is actually the antidote to our helplessness. That's because the
way we explain a trying situation can either catapult us into depres-
sion or bolster our resilience.

Dr. Martin Seligman states in his book *Learned Optimism* that changing the explanation of an event can lift our mood and help us face the future with feelings of hope and competence. "Finding temporary and specific causes of misfortune is the art of hope: Temporary causes limit helplessness in time, and specific causes limit our helplessness to the original situation." As parents, this is something we urgently need to learn—how to think about situations as temporary and specifically caused.

To explain our disastrous dinner in an optimistic way, for instance, I would point out that the restaurant was very dark and crowded, and the waiters weren't supportive to families. Understandably, the children reacted to the noise, the dimness, and the long wait for food. Rather than being at fault, the parents were patient and endlessly creative. More importantly, I would state that this challenging hour was an insignificant event in the big picture, but one that the parents could learn from to make future dinners more enjoyable.

The next time, we ate out together at a restaurant with a bright open patio, where the tables were well spaced and noise was low. The children ate happily, and we stayed after dinner relaxing and enjoying our time together. Who knows whether my assumptions were right about the change in ambiance? My point is, blaming the bad time on the environment makes us feel less helpless and relieves us of blame. Making the explanation revolve around a temporary and very specific situation makes an hour just an hour, with no implications for the future.

We can endure almost anything for an hour, and the idea that we only need to parent one hour at a time is one of the best attitudes we can hold. It helps us to let go of setbacks, hold on to optimism, and teach positive outlooks to our children. We owe it to our kids to see life as hopeful and believe in our abilities to handle obstacles, even when we feel helpless. Kids catch our positive thoughts, especially when we stay aware of how important it is for us to believe in them and in ourselves.

Analyze your attitudes when you're overwhelmed by your child's behavior. Do you ascribe the upset to problems in the moment, or picture yourself continuing to struggle with your child into the future?

Kids Reflect Positive Thoughts

Life mirrors my every thought. As I keep my thoughts positive, life brings to me only good experiences. As I say yes to life, life says yes to me.

LOUISE HAY

When they were exhausted from an impossible situation with one of their kids, Paula and her husband, Dave, had a game they sometimes played. They took turns asserting that child's good qualities. "She plays the piano with such great concentration and beauty." "She really likes to entertain the family." "She has such wonderful fantasies in her play." Ultimately, they would start laughing, since their positive comments had nothing to do with the recent misbehavior. Searching for happy things to say was an exercise in restoring a positive image of their child.

When a child is acting up, our society encourages people to worry about whether the behavior is part of a bigger problem—a disorder, a psychological issue, a disability. But it doesn't usually help to see our child's behavior in this drastic light—in fact, doing so can cause children to doubt themselves. Since children absorb a parent's thoughts like a sponge soaks up water, Paula and Dave played the game to let go of their negative perspective and start fresh.

When parents are frustrated by a child's behavior, I often ask them to stop and think for a moment what it would be like if their spouse or best friend thought of them as a problem. People usually cringe, imagining how it would feel to pick up on a loved one's dissatisfaction.

In *You Can Be Happy No Matter What*, Dr. Richard Carlson advises us that we can solve problems productively by not ruminating on them. He describes the "snowball effect"—we perceive something as a problem, and our attention to it causes it to grow in our minds and affect those around us. He points out that not thinking about another person's problems is an instantaneous way to improve a marriage. The process of not focusing on problems works beautifully in a marriage or relationship. He reports that his clients have often perfected "the art of bad marriage in their heads—they had gone over and over the same things in an attempt to straighten each other out. What will help is to increase the positive feeling state in ourselves by not focusing on problems."

The flip side of recognizing that negative feelings hurt a relationship is recognizing how much positive thoughts help. I have learned over the years that one of the best things I can do with my concern over a child is to concentrate on her wonderful qualities. This doesn't mean I forget about the problem behavior. However, I shift my focus to include all the times the problem doesn't occur and to pay attention to other facets of the child's personality. I don't want the child to think of herself as a problem. Holding the attitude that children react to my thoughts keeps me aware of my own ruminations.

One day I was puzzling over a four-year-old boy's habit of screaming when he wanted something, rather than asking a teacher. I talked to the teachers about various ways of responding. A couple of days later, he came and sat on my lap. A warm feeling grew between us, and we sat together for forty-five minutes or more. I started noticing how sweet and affectionate he was. What a great smile. As I thought about these things, he looked up and smiled or patted me. I could see that he was taking in my happy thoughts about him. As his teachers made friends with him, they noticed his screaming decreased. Suddenly, he was basking in positive attention and didn't need to yell in order to get it. His screaming didn't vanish, but he slowly learned that he could talk to his teachers.

Children aren't conscious of their special qualities, nor do they necessarily have names for them. By showing that we notice and respond favorably to their traits, we are teaching them what their strengths are.

A teacher told me recently that she often tells a child how his positive quality affects her. She might say, "I saw how brave you were when someone called you a name today, and you didn't say something nasty back. Your courage made me feel strong, too."

Children's strengths will affect others throughout their lives. It's our job to notice that they kept trying when something proved hard for them, or that they refrained from making a poor choice. Making them aware of their developing strengths helps them approach life with confidence and trust.

Rephrasing what we see as a child's weak areas can help change our perspective.

Circle the rephrased adjectives that describe your child:

Shy	**Slow to warm up**
Fearful	**Careful**
Bossy	**Knows his own mind, likes to lead**
Stubborn	**Determined, persevering**
Demands attention	**Able to communicate needs**
Clingy	**Likes to connect**
Naughty	**Spontaneous**
Rigid	**High sense of order**
Selfish	**Values possessions**
Loud	**Expressive**

The World Needs
Our Children's Gifts

Real education consists of drawing the best
out of yourself.

GANDHI

One of the most authoritative voices in the English-speaking world
belongs to actor James Earl Jones, famous for his many film roles as
well as for the voices of Darth Vader in *Star Wars* and King Mufasa in
The Lion King. Jones is considered by many to be one of the greatest
actors of the twentieth century. Yet the fact that he can use his voice
to communicate at all results from a miracle of positive thinking on
the part of one adult in his life.

From the time James was six years old until he reached the age of
fifteen, he was almost entirely mute. Born in Mississippi, James was
raised by his grandparents after being abandoned by both his father
and mother shortly after his birth. Stress about his family's move to
Michigan caused James to start stuttering. Then fear of stuttering
made him afraid to talk. His grandparents never chastised him for not
speaking, but his grandfather lamented not hearing James' voice
because it had always been so beautiful.

At school, James' teachers accepted his self-imposed limitations,
allowing him to communicate what he learned in written form. His
potential acting abilities could have been lost to the world if it had not
been for his tenth-grade English teacher, Donald E. Crouch. Crouch
introduced James to literature—Shakespeare, Emerson, and

Longfellow. James was moved to write poetry himself and on tasting grapefruit for the first time, crafted a poem based on the cadence and rhythm of Longfellow's poem *Hiawatha*. Delighted to learn that James was writing poetry, Mr. Crouch pointed out that the way to prove that the poem about grapefruit was really his own was to read it in front of the class. Crouch's approach was subtle. He didn't pressure James or tell him he *should* read the poem. He sympathized with his student, telling him that he knew how painful it was for him to talk and that he wouldn't require it. However, he saw that James' love of words was one of his strengths, and he appealed to that passion in order to help him overcome his weakness.

James believed Crouch's edict that a poet should read his own words aloud and agreed to read the poem. However, the day he stood in front of the class to read his grapefruit poem, his body began to shake, and he recalls that he pushed the words "from the bottom of my soul." Everyone, including James and his teacher, was amazed that when he read from his page he never stuttered once. "Basically, he tricked me into speaking," Jones remembers.

In the process, they both discovered that James, like many stutterers, could read a script perfectly. "Aha," the teacher exclaimed. "We will now use this to recapture your ability to speak." Under Crouch's tutelage, James became the school speaking champion and the valedictorian of his class. That was how the world began to benefit from James' talents.

What a privilege it is to be the person in a child's life who looks past his weaknesses to see the gifts that will become gateways for new development. That doesn't mean ignoring areas where our children need help. We just need to emphasize their natural abilities and interests. If no one notices what they love, children may never connect with their passions and work on expanding them. Believing that our children's strengths are far more important than their weaknesses is one of the best attitudes we can hold.

In fifth and sixth grade, I had one of those teachers who changes a child's life: Anne Candia. She saw each child in our class as possessing a unique gift. She encouraged me in writing, and, although I had been extremely shy, I came to love reading my writing to the class. She encouraged others in singing, others in sports. Her fascination with what we did well helped us not to think about what we couldn't do. It was as if our teacher was determined that each of us would contribute our strengths to the world. She trusted in our futures, even when we were at our worst, and put all her effort into helping us trust ourselves.

Can you remember a parent or teacher who believed in you, even when you were failing or refusing to believe in yourself? What words would he or she have used to describe you?

Substitute Trust for Fear

Do your best. Don't worry, be happy.

MEHER BABA

The call came late at night. "Don't get stressed," my twenty-six-year-old daughter warned on the phone. My heart started racing, but I didn't respond. "I can only tell you what's going on here if you promise not to worry."

"What's the alternative?" I thought to myself. My daughter is 10,000 miles away from home, studying in Russia, and she won't confide in me unless I stay calm.

"That's fine, honey," I said in a calm voice. "I want to hear what's going on. I was wondering why we hadn't heard from you."

"They may not be showing it on the news yet in the U.S., but the whole city of Moscow is in crisis," she said quickly, as if she might have to hang up any minute. "Have you heard of the banking crisis?" I said that I had. "Well, it's much worse here than the American media might be presenting it. People are panicking. You can't get dollars out of the bank, so I can't get any money. I'm figuring out what to do."

"Come home!" I wanted to shout. But I was afraid that might reveal my frenzied state of mind. Instead I took a breath and asked, "What do you plan to do?"

In this situation, I wanted to give her strength by demonstrating my faith in her decisions, rather than worry her with my concerns. Besides, she might hang up if I started crying. In order to remain calm, I began to concentrate on all the ways my daughter was showing her competence. She is responsible, I told myself, and incredibly determined. She is strong.

I learned this technique of concentrating on her abilities when she was about three. She used to cry and cling to my leg like a crab when I first brought her to preschool. The teacher said it would help her if I didn't worry. I wondered if the teacher knew that I was an inveterate worrier, or if she said this to all the parents. I always thought worrying was a way to protect your kids from harm. But the teacher's vision opened my mind to new possibilities.

I began to picture worry as a kind of static that kids can pick up on. So when I left the preschool classroom I forced myself to imagine my daughter having a great time. She loves other kids, I told myself. She wants to learn. She is terribly determined. I was surprised to find that if I focused on my daughter's capacity to cope, rather than on the tears, we both did better. Thinking about her natural abilities to cope bolstered mine.

My Russian story had a satisfying ending. My daughter came home a happy and even more confident person. But between that call and the time she walked off the plane, I worked hard to trust rather than fear.

Worrying isn't wrong, but it does rob us of energy. Before our children are adults, we still can assess the risks of places they want to go and set limits. But many of the challenges our children face come unexpectedly, and worrying doesn't give us the ability to control their lives. Concentrating on their coping skills can give us more peace of mind and help them to trust themselves.

A woman in her thirties talked to me one day about her father's lack of worry and how much it helped her development. "My dad just never worried about us," she said proudly. "It wasn't that we never had crises or made mistakes. He just always had faith that we would deal with things and be fine." She felt that his unshakable faith in her gave her confidence in herself and the competence to handle what life dishes out. She is one of the most confident young women I've ever met!

Living in today's world promises to challenge our children to hold every kind of fear and doubt. One of the best things we can do for them and ourselves is to say, "Worry will rob you of life's joy. I believe in you and know you can do it!"

Imagine that you are starting a new job soon or leaving for a trip to a new place. How will it feel if your best friend worries about you and fills you with apprehensive advice? How would your reaction change if your friend acted as if she trusted your abilities to handle the challenges involved? Notice how children react when adults caution them.

CHAPTER 3

Focus on Feelings

Nurture Joy

We can enhance joy deliberately by not taking joy for
granted, but rather permitting ourselves to delight in a
joyful child. . . . We do know that joy grows in children
when it is reinforced.

DR. VERENA KAST

When my one-year-old grandson is happy, he claps his hands or pats
my arm. Sometimes he just smiles, throwing back his head and shut-
ting his eyes. Watching him, I try to join him. The source of his joy is
often apparent—the sifting sand in his fingers, the pried lid of a small
metal box, or the rhythm of the music that flows from the stereo. I've
also realized that he doesn't need such entertainment to find happiness. It's woven through him.

My wish is that his capacity for joy will expand rather than diminish
with time. But in general, as we watch children grow, many of them
seem to lose this capacity. What a tragedy! What are the skills for helping children retain this jubilant feeling? As a teacher, I have acquired
techniques for helping a child with anger, sadness, and frustration. But
encouraging a child's joy was never addressed in my training.

Dr. Verena Kast, one of the rare psychologists to study positive
emotions, recommends learning about joy by tapping into our childhood memories of happiness. She says that asking ourselves what
brought us delight when we were young helps us to discover happiness in our lives now. This approach is a departure from the emphasis
our society places on learning about early wounds. What would our

childhoods have been like if people had dedicated themselves to making us more joyous?

I can't recall joy being a goal in life as I was growing up. When people talked to me about my potential, it was always in terms of attributes that would help me "make it" in the world. For me, the moments of intense happiness were secret: discovering blue lupine and tiny wild strawberries as I walked on a hill, trying to beat my father in a footrace, hitting a tether ball with all my might. I wonder if my parents noticed how happy those experiences made me.

Today I observe parents noticing their children's joyful moments and seeking them out. At our school, busy parents sometimes take the long path through our butterfly garden to observe a rosebush in bloom or look for tadpoles in the pond. These parents have observed the transformation that occurs when a child notices something that interests her.

However, as children get older, our society also teaches them that joy occurs when they get what they want—whether it be a new toy, a new outfit, or being on the winning side in a baseball game. If good feeling is dependent on attainment, then the law of averages dictates that our children will be joyless at least some portion of the time. Is happiness that is derived from getting what we want fulfilling?

Many parents are able to help children seek joy even when life is challenging. When four-year-old Sam's family moved, he had a hard time adjusting. He showed signs of stress, and his mom and dad worked hard to support him. But his parents were concentrated not just on coping, but also on activities that brought an abundance of good feeling. They noticed Sam liked to look at clouds. One night when they looked out the window at a cloud formation, Sam said, "Mom, someday I want to start a cloud museum. That way everyone can come and see the most beautiful clouds." His mother delighted in his sense of wonder. She and Sam started taking photographs of clouds and putting them in albums. Sam's mother helped him to learn that joy is waiting for him at even the hardest times, if he remembers to turn toward it.

The ability to access a positive flow of emotion is a gift that can last a lifetime. But embracing joy doesn't mean we should dismiss children's troubling feelings, such as anger or fear. As we learn to focus on feelings, we can help our children begin to understand all their emotions and handle them with care.

Recall what adults told you about joy as a child. Was it portrayed as a feeling you had to contain? Imagine a time when you felt happy as a child. How did you express joy? How do you experience it now? How do you react when your child feels elated?

Don't Dismiss Their Fears

It didn't work to tell my four-year-old son, "Monsters aren't real." He couldn't understand the idea of unreality. I sympathized with his fear and told him I felt that way as a kid. I gave him a squirt bottle to spray monsters at night. He loved it.

TIM, FATHER OF TWO

Over one lunchtime, my then four-year-old daughter's perspective toward preschool took a 180-degree turn. In the morning Mari loved school, as she had for the last year. After lunch, she never wanted to go back. I had called to tell the teacher I was going to be a few minutes behind schedule—no big deal, since my daughter loved to stay late. But this time she heard the teacher's words as, "Your mom isn't coming back." In her mind, my daughter tacked on the word "ever." In that moment, the image that I was never coming back was imprinted indelibly on her mind. She felt traumatized, and on the way home from school that's all she talked about.

I have to admit that over the next few days, I started going crazy. No matter how many times I explained that she had misunderstood the teacher when she was explaining I was late, the fearful image gripped her.

As I have seen many times, terror takes off like a raging fire in a sensitive child's mind. No rational explanation seems to put it out. Therapist Cecilia Soares of Walnut Creek, California, points out, "It's very difficult for children to use reasoning with their fears. That's what makes their anxieties more primitive and intense. Saying 'there's nothing to be afraid of' doesn't connect with their feelings. They need soothing. They want to hear that you will make things safe."

A professional counselor and friend had advised me not to pull Mari out of school because she had gotten scared, but to help her work through the fear. That way she would develop faith in her abilities to cope. Keeping her home would reinforce her fear that it's dangerous to go out into the world because mom might not come back. When we gently encourage children to find ways to express their fears and deal with them, we help them discover their courage and resilience.

I thought about my childhood anxiety about my mother not coming back and the comfort I would have liked. Instead of telling Mari there was nothing to be afraid of, I validated her feelings, telling her that I sometimes had the same fears when I was her age. If my mom was late, I would cry and cry. Over time, I understood that my mother did come back. I told Mari I loved her and I would always come back. "Do you believe that?" I asked. She said she did, but she was still afraid. I suggested she tell herself, "My mother loves me, and she always comes back," at school during the morning. She tried repeating that phrase and found it helped her. I felt a little less crazy. Affirmations like this aren't the same as dismissing fear or offering a rational explanation. They are words designed to program our subconscious and our emotions in positive ways. Gradually Mari's fear diminished, and when she went to kindergarten, she couldn't wait to get to school. Later, psychologist Wendy Ritchey and I coauthored a book called *I Think I Can I Know I Can*, about helping children to have positive self-talk.

Tuning in to our children's fears by remembering the times we were afraid as children is one of the best things we can do. Saying we're afraid now, as adults, could make them feel insecure, but knowing that we were once fearful of the same things shows children that they can always confide their anxieties in us. But often our children don't know what's troubling them and act out their distress in ways we don't understand. Getting upset at them for the "bad behavior" spurred by inner turmoil doesn't work. We need to let go of our mental constructs about the way they should be acting, when fears persist, and enter into our own feeling realm in order to understand.

Record some of the fears that haunted you as a child. How did adults respond to them? If you had a persistent fear, what approach would have helped you feel safe?

I Felt That Way Once

What finally helped me most was actually putting
myself in my children's shoes. I asked myself, "Suppose
I were a child who was tired, hot, or bored? And suppose I wanted that all-important grownup in my life to
know what I was feeling?"

ADELE FABER AND ELAINE MAZLISH

Sue and Luis couldn't understand their four-year-old son Jacob's
behavior. Lately he had been throwing tantrums for no apparent
reason. If his twin sister sang in the car, he went to pieces. If he got
frustrated with a toy at home, he started screaming.

The child-rearing books they read recommended ignoring tantrums.
But Sue and Luis found that the more they tried to tune out Jacob's
outbursts, the more frequent and ferocious they became. Was his defi-
ance a way of getting back at them for something? How could they
cope with this strange behavior? That's when they came to see me.

I asked them if there was any new stress in their family life.
Children often express their strain through increased upset or waking
at night. They said nothing was different at home. I could see that
struggling to intellectually understand Jacob was frustrating them.

I asked if either of them could think of times when their emotions
felt out of control, either now or when they were kids. Sue said she
felt that way on days when she was overwhelmed with work. I asked
if she liked Luis to ignore her at those times. "I would be furious," she
said emphatically. "I would probably feel abandoned, like he didn't

care." She thought for a moment. "What I want is for Luis to stay calm. I don't want him to get angry about me being emotionally over-wrought."

Then, thinking about wanting Luis to stay calm, Sue said, "I don't know why I've gotten so angry about Jacob's feelings and taken them so personally. He must feel terrible about us ignoring him." Empathizing with her son, she suddenly remembered that they had, indeed, had a new stress in their family. Her grandfather was sick, and she had to be at the nursing home a lot. "Jacob must be upset because I'm gone so much and I'm so stressed about my grandfather when I'm home. He doesn't know how to tell me."

I thought that Sue's awareness that she didn't want Luis to ignore her or be "upset by her upset" offered profound insight. When we're emotionally overwhelmed, we don't want others to get agitated or indignant. We need their calm support. "Ignoring" doesn't mean pretending the person isn't there; it has more to do with not getting angry or caving in to demands. Our need to fix our child's outburst can add our negative energy to his.

When we're agitated by our child's upset, it's also easy to imagine negative explanations that have nothing to do with reality. When we have a tough time consoling our new baby, we may think she's mad at us or that we're incompetent. When a child screams to have his own way, we may fear we're raising a monster. Remembering the times when we've been crazily tired or disappointed about not getting something can give us a more reassuring and realistic picture.

It sounds simple, but sometimes the most straightforward approach proves the most profound. What helps at any age is just to have someone notice, "I see you're sad (or angry or frustrated)," without any judgment.

Two weeks later, Sue told me that she had spoken to Jacob about being gone so much. They're also spending more time together. "I'm not worried anymore," Sue said with a smile. "He's not throwing as many tantrums." Her lack of worry is also part of the cure. She's calmer.

Our emotional links to our children give us the unique sensitivity to effectively support them. When we're connected, our very presence has the power to make them feel safe. We do that best when we remember the force of their love and put consistent effort into protecting that connection.

Write about a time as a child when an adult helped you to overcome an upset. What was it in the adult's manner that helped you recover your sense of balance?

My Children Love Me So Much

**My mother was the making of me. She was so true
and so sure of me. I felt I had someone I must not
disappoint. The memory of my mother will always be
a blessing to me.**

THOMAS A. EDISON

I went one evening to hear Hillary Clinton speak about children when
her book *It Takes a Village* was released. She was knowledgeable,
inspiring, and obviously deeply concerned about the world's children.
But the story I will never forget was the one she told about her own
child, Chelsea. When Chelsea was about eight, the family went to
church on Mother's Day in Little Rock, Arkansas. The minister asked
each of the children in the congregation, "If you could give your
mother anything, what would it be?" One child said a beautiful purple
dress, another said jewels. When it was Chelsea's turn, she said she
wanted to give her mother life insurance. Hillary smiled appreciatively
at Chelsea, but wondered what her daughter had in mind. On the way
home, she asked in a kindly, inquiring way why her daughter wanted
to give her life insurance. "Because I love you so much, I never want
you to die," said Chelsea. Hillary was stunned and shared the insight
with us she had gleaned that Mother's Day morning. "We could never
imagine how much our children love us and how crucial we are in
their lives, but we have to try."

This story reminds me of how wonderful it is when parents don't
underestimate their children's feelings of attachment to them. John

Bowlby was one of the first psychologists to establish that strong attachments provide a child with "a secure base." A mother goes to work in the morning and leaves her baby with someone else—a caregiver the child hopefully learns to love. But the mother may worry that her baby won't fly into her arms when she picks her up that afternoon. Separation and reunion are a big deal and spur complex emotions, even as a child grows older. I've known a secure eight year old to wet her pants when her mother goes away overnight. Part of knowing how much our child loves us is paying close attention to that separation process and helping it go well.

Like Hillary Clinton, many parents have jobs or roles that require them to be away from their children for days at a time. Those children might like to give their parents life insurance. The thought that a parent might not come back can be lurking in their minds even if they don't show it. Mothers and fathers who keep their children's overwhelming feelings of attachment in their awareness don't dismiss their strong feelings by saying things like, "You won't even notice that I'm gone." I don't know how Hillary Clinton helped Chelsea cope with her times away, but I am privileged to see how many parents I know handle these separations in sensitive ways.

My friend Mary Jane made a "Mama chart" for her daughter with a square for every day she would be gone on her business trip. Daddy Don helped Ana color in the square for that day, and they would count the days until she came home. I watched Mary Jane pick Ana up one day at school as she came back from a trip. On that particular day, Ana turned away and wouldn't look at her. Mary Jane commented that Ana was angry. I told her how wonderful I thought it was that she knew Ana's anger was part of loving her. "Why wouldn't she be angry?" Mary Jane asked. "The most important person in her world left her. She adores her dad, but it's really hard for her when I'm gone and I'm very aware of that." That's why she makes her homecomings special.

One day I couldn't help but stop to watch another reunion: a mother kneeling in her good suit on one knee in the hallway of her son's preschool. Her son was coming from the other end of the hall. She held out her arms, and her voice sounded as if she hadn't seen him for a month, though it was actually just since that morning. "I missed you so much!" she said, embracing him. Her words and body language showed him that she understood that being away from her for a whole day could feel like a month. His huge adoring smile made my day.

What were the situations that made you feel connected to your parents? Were there things they did or didn't do that caused you to shut them out or feel clingy and insecure?

PART II

The
BeST
THiNGs
PaReNTS
DO

Our next step is exploring the helpful things parents actually do. Where do we hear about the remarkable progress parents have made in recent generations? Today's parents are bombarded with more information about child psychology and development than they can possibly process, yet they do a surprisingly good job of integrating information and "walking all the talk" that they receive. Why do we ignore how often today's parents succeed in acting according to the best of their ability and knowledge? Without documenting the countless things parents do well, we have no model of good parenting.

The stories in this chapter don't reflect the lives of "all-knowing" parents who exercise their best awareness all the time. They are based on tales of real people—myself included—making mistakes; gaining insight; learning from observations, discussions, and reading; taking classes; remembering what it's like to be a child; and following their intuition.

As you read these situations, I hope you will think of your own ideas about the best things parents do, and especially the things you do when you are at your best. I also hope you won't compare yourself to these people, except to identify with their feelings and their willingness to experiment and learn. We each have our own path when it comes to relating to children, and the things we actually do help create our wisdom.

As the ancient saying attributed to Lao-Tzu goes, "A journey of a thousand miles begins with but a single step." Each of the steps we take paves the way for others to walk with wisdom and open themselves to new learning.

CHAPTER 4

Bring Out Their Best

Teach Self-Sufficiency

Give a man a fish, and you feed him for a day. Teach a
man to fish, and you feed him for a lifetime.

CHINESE PROVERB

Years ago a reporter called to interview me from Florida. She had
read somewhere that my twelve-year-old daughter did her own laundry, and she wondered how a young girl managed such a big responsibility. I felt a little embarrassed. My daughter had been washing her
clothes for several years (my son had, too). If the reporter thought
twelve was too young to launder, what about eight or nine? I reassured her that my daughter washed her clothes with competence.
Then she moved to the heart of the issue. "Isn't it the mom's job to do
the laundry?" she asked, in a sweet but confused tone. "I have a daughter, and doing her clothes is one of the ways I nurture her." Gulp!

Thinking about it, I realized the reporter and I were seeing love and
nurturance in different ways. Doing someone's laundry is nurturing—
unless you keep doing it after they are capable, and they are helpless
to wash their own T-shirt and shorts. One of the ways I nurtured my
children was to make them feel capable of caring for themselves. I
wanted them to feel confident and self-sufficient when they left home.
In college, my kids encountered people who had never learned to
wash clothes or cook a meal. Their embarrassment made them feel
too old to learn.

A wise schoolteacher once told me that the secret of motivating
children to do practical tasks is to teach them while the skill is chal-

lenging. A four year old begs to sweep the floor and wash the table. An eight year old still likes to learn about laundry. So I tried to start teaching my kids these chores while they still wanted to learn.

I was motivated by the realization as a young adult that I hadn't acquired enough skills before leaving home, and I felt lacking. My mother showed love by doing things for me. I have a friend whose mother still drew her bath when she was a teenager, and she had a hard transition to the adult world, too.

Almost every fairy tale revolves around the symbolic question, "Will I be self-sufficient enough to go out into the world?" Deep inside, children really appreciate everything they learn about caring for themselves, because being able to do everything for oneself is the core of self-sufficiency. That's why kids love *Pippi Longstocking*, the story of a little girl who lives by herself and knows how to do everything.

There is a famous story in educational circles that illustrates children's gratitude for learning self-sufficiency. When Dr. Maria Montessori, the great Italian educator, first opened her school for tenement children, she was constantly surprised by their profound desire to learn practical skills. Since they always had runny noses, she decided to teach her students the fine points of discreetly blowing one's nose. The children were silent as they watched, and then they shocked her by bursting into applause. They had been ridiculed for their runny noses, but no one had demonstrated how to clean them.

I would definitely put "blowing nose" on the top of my list of skills for children to acquire in life. What about your list? Since it feels as if each stage will last forever, it helps to occasionally switch perspectives and picture your child going out the door with a suitcase to college or some other adventure at seventeen. What are the things that you want him to know? What practical skills should she have? Hold this image so you can plan how to teach your child self-sufficiency well in advance.

We can't teach our children everything before they leave home. But we can train them to learn the practical life skills they will need to feel confident. We can expect them to become capable contributors to our homes and show them how much we appreciate their efforts to make things run smoothly.

Make a list of all the things you wish you had learned before leaving home.
What do you want your child to know by the age of eighteen?
How can you start working toward those goals now?

Hold High Expectations

It's a funny thing about life; if you refuse to accept anything but the best, you often get it.

SOMERSET MAUGHAM

Lynn was working as an exotic dancer when she first met her neighbor's daughters. She thought they were cute but completely out of control. The oldest had just told her kindergarten teacher to "F— off! You die!" The young girls lived next door with their father, and she would hear them fighting with each other and throwing fits. He had just received sole custody, and Lynn felt sorry for the girls because they seemed to live in a world without expectations or structure. She knew how scary it is for a child to have to keep testing to find out the limits. The girls got chickenpox, and their father had no one to care for them while he worked. "I worked nights, so I thought why not try being with kids during the day?" Lynn found she had a knack for creating order and happiness out of chaos.

Soon Lynn had the girls helping to keep the house neat, following rules, and sitting on "time-out" when they didn't listen or hurt each other. "No one expected much of the girls, and it had been fine for them to swear and show disrespect to adults. I changed all that by seeing them as capable helpers." The girls appreciated the gentle, consistent structure Lynn imposed. Their father was amazed to come home to an immaculate apartment at the end of a day and find the girls cuddled up reading a story with his neighbor.

In time, Lynn fell in love with the man and they married, and Lynn left her dancing job, creating an even firmer foundation for the girls. The couple had another baby of their own, and suddenly Lynn was the mother of three. How does she cope? The secret is expecting everyone to help. She creates a structure that makes their household run with such cooperation that not all the work falls on her. The older girls are now in junior high and elementary school, and they have chore charts that outline what needs to be done before and after school. The charts remind them of self-care tasks like putting dirty clothes in the hamper, bathing, and making their own lunches. In addition, each girl has jobs that help the whole house run efficiently, such as taking out the garbage, setting the table, and doing dishes. The littlest girl is in preschool; she is expected to set the table and help with cooking.

"Sometimes the girls ask me why they have to do chores when few of their friends do. I tell them I can't do everything around the house or I'll be mad all the time. Other people might be afraid to ask their kids to help for fear they'll be resentful, but I would feel lacking as a parent if I didn't. It's hard for me to maintain the consistency, but I know that our regularity gives them internal structure. I love seeing how capable they are. It's great! They feel confident to do anything. One of them just organized a surprise party for a friend."

The girls are also allowed to do extra-credit jobs. If they do, they can pick a fun adventure for the family, like going to a restaurant of their choice.

From my perspective, Lynn has provided just the right framework for her daughters. In a study of discipline in the 1960s, Dr. Diana Baumrind of U.C. Berkeley found that children whose parents consistently hold high expectations and firm limits for them develop into more self-confident, self-reliant people.

We don't have to be organizational wizards like Lynn to make a child feel competent. A structured household just consists of clear limits, predictable routines, and taking the time to teach everyone to contribute. We can start with the things they want to do for themselves, no matter how inept they seem, since the desire "to do" lies at the heart of accomplishment.

Break down household tasks into steps to help children learn them more easily.

What are the steps of setting a table?

Folding a towel?

Making a bed?

Sweeping a floor?

Ignite the Fire of Accomplishment

People's confidence grows as they attempt and complete tasks. Success increases confidence; failure diminishes it . . . the messages individuals receive from others can powerfully influence their development.

FRANK PAJARES

When I want to illustrate how a child develops an "I can do!" attitude, I always think of Johnny's father, Fred.

When Johnny was about eight, he saw a high-school production of *Fiddler on the Roof*. Since he was taking violin lessons, he was captivated by the man who sat on the roof playing the violin and told his father that he wished that he could have a roof to play on. Fred took him seriously, and together they gathered scrap wood to build him a "roof." But how do you make a roof without a house? So they also constructed a six-foot tower with a ladder to a flat plywood roof. Johnny was absolutely thrilled to sit there and play his tunes. Johnny didn't grow up to become a violinist, but his confidence in his ability to accomplish what he set out to do led him to find his own money to attend medical school and become a doctor, who plays the violin for pleasure.

The great Sufi teacher Inayat Khan once wrote, "Accomplishment is more valuable than what is accomplished. For instance, if a person has loosened a knot in a string, apparently he has not gained anything, the time has been spent on a very small thing. And yet the action of completing it is useful, he has built something in his spirit that will be useful to him when he wants to accomplish great works."

Inayat Khan emphasizes the action of completion as having special significance. Yet today we often don't consider the importance to children of finishing what they start. A child starts to work on a puzzle and leaves it when it gets hard. In the middle of setting the table, a child answers the phone and forgets about his task. A girl says she wants to draw a unicorn, but two minutes later she crumples the paper up because her first attempt didn't meet her satisfaction. Perhaps Johnny even balked at all the cutting and hammering and wanted to run off to play, but his father helped him to keep working until they were finished.

Having self-efficacy means we have confidence in our "power to produce the desired effect." That power is different from self-esteem, or feeling good about oneself. Bolstering children's sense of capability influences them to evaluate themselves more positively. Adults can enhance their accomplishments by helping them to see things to completion. Sometimes children grow frustrated when they are building with blocks or drawing, because they don't have the skill to make the product according to their internal image. If an adult notices, she can help by problem solving with the child to see how she could accomplish what she set out to do. Doing it for her won't help build an internal spirit of accomplishment, but helping her see the task to completion will. It can be challenging when a child cries and wants to give up. But if we regard her frustration as positive and say, "You want to make it just right, don't you?" she will be more apt to try to complete that and other projects.

Millie's daughter just began junior high—a time when interests often get spread in many directions. "Whenever I see her get frustrated on a project, I offer to help her to finish it. I never had the feeling growing up that I could do anything, and I want her to have that confidence. Recently, she had the idea that she could compose songs for a book report and videotape herself singing them. I don't think she realized what a big idea it was, but I helped her figure out the notes and make the videotape. It was quite an undertaking, but it worked out and she presented it."

The saying, "It's attitude not aptitude that determines your altitude," expresses the fact that what we believe about ourselves is even more important than our inherent abilities and talents. Many geniuses never achieve their dreams or contribute to the world; it's the belief that we are capable and can live out our ideals that keeps us feeling fulfilled in life.

Can you think of a project that you were proud you completed as a child? How did that sense of accomplishment feel?

Initiate Ideals

You must work—we must all work—to make the world worthy of its children.

PABLO CASALS

When Sarah's son Ian started calling his friends names like "Stupid" and "Baby" at the age of four, she decided that there was enough name calling in the world, and she didn't want her son to contribute to it. Other parents reassured her that name calling is a favorite four-year-old activity. Sarah agreed that communicating anger in a civilized way proves challenging for all four year olds. But as a former teacher she had observed that calling people foul names, instead of talking out a conflict, isn't a phase. "I know that calling someone a 'poo-poo head' at four sounds harmless, and saying it's not okay might seem silly. But I've seen that the names get worse once the habit starts, and it can get really ugly in elementary school and adolescence." Sarah is convinced that the name calling leads to scapegoating and bullying.

She decided that treating others respectfully was a value she wanted to uphold in her family. Sarah talked to Ian, telling him that it was fine for him to say, "I'm angry at you," or "Don't grab my toy." But she wouldn't allow name calling because it hurts others' feelings. He would feel bad if someone shouted a mean name at him. They role-played situations that made him angry with other kids at school, discussing ways he could assert himself without name calling. In spite of these explanations, Ian did what his friends did.

Sarah worried if being strict with Ian about the name calling was unreasonable or making the situation worse. Should she give up? Instead, she decided she felt so strongly about respect that she would take a different, more forceful tack. She told Ian that, when they were on a play date at one of his friends' houses, if he called his friend a name, she would enforce a consequence, taking him home immediately. This was socially risky business for Sarah! The hostess, looking forward to visiting with her, might not sympathize with her decision to leave a few minutes after she arrived. But Sarah was determined. "It only took about three abrupt departures for Ian to get the message. He dropped the habit of calling names completely." When others observed Sarah's success, they changed their views and started prohibiting name calling, too. Everyone noticed how much more nicely the children played. In her circle of friends, the little ripple Sarah started turned into a wave.

Today Ian is eight and well liked by his friends. Sarah feels a sense of fulfillment that the value of treating others respectfully has become an integral part of his relationships. "Ian and his friends don't put each other down. They show that disrespecting others doesn't have to be the norm." It's difficult to uphold an ideal like not calling names, when our culture has become so steeped in using insults as a major source of humor. Our media project the attitude that the ability to verbally duel proves that someone is cool. Sarah admits that she has to be absolutely consistent about not allowing that mentality in her house, since it's such a pervasive part of our culture.

One of the best perspectives we can hold as parents is to believe that what we do and what our children do matter in the grand scheme of things. The process begins with not letting ourselves off the hook where honesty or kindness is concerned. Studies also show that when parents take a people-oriented approach, as Sarah did ("Calling names hurts feelings.") rather than enforcing a rule ("Calling names is wrong!), children grow more empathetic—an essential quality in moral development.

Our families are the microcosm where high ideals are born. As Pablo Casals says in the quote introducing this chapter, we must all work to make the world a better place. It's easy to point fingers at others for their lack of values. But our real work is taking a strong stance ourselves and letting our children know why.

When we demonstrate that virtues like honesty, respect for others, kindness, or loyalty aren't just words to us—that we are willing to take a stand on those ideals—our children are more apt to initiate them in their interactions. Catching them in their attempts to be kind and considerate encourages them to adopt those values as their own.

Make a list of five values that you want your children to learn. How do you model them in your own life?

Catch Them in Acts of Kindness

Kindness can become its own motive. We are made kind by being kind.

ERIC HOFFER

My two-and-a-half-year-old grandson, Malachi, drives his plastic fire engine over to the couch where my husband and I are reading to his one-and-a-half-year-old sister, Lila. He carefully parks, hangs his firefighter's hat on the edge of the coffee table, and snuggles in to hear the story. Almost as quickly, Lila silently slips off the couch, mounts the fire engine, and propels herself across the room. Malachi leaps off the couch and tackles her, trying to lift her off the engine by her neck. We rush to remove his hands from Lila's craned neck, while she continues to drive, shouting, "Mine!" Finally we lift him up and talk to him about his sister having a peaceful turn with the fire engine. He isn't convinced, but we succeed in distracting him with some face paints. When his parents return, he has a design on his cheek and—how timely!— they want to discuss remedies for sibling fighting.

As grandparent babysitters, we hadn't prevented conflict, so my suggestion includes the reminder that brothers and sisters fighting is normal. In fact, it's one of the ways that children learn to negotiate with others. I advised that the most powerful tool for promoting positive interaction is noticing and commenting on Malachi and Lila's acts of kindness and positive interaction with each other. I always try to comment on their harmonious play and the times when they use words instead of fists to settle a dispute. Giving attention to their attempts to interact peacefully raises the chances that they will try the same techniques again. Research also shows that the more times a child acts kind or helpful, the more he will want to do so in the future. It's a matter of training ourselves to notice the positive.

On the surface, this task sounds easy, but it can be difficult to do systematically. When children play nicely, we tend not to notice. Sometimes their positive actions may also be too quick for us to reinforce. And, when disputes occur, it's tempting to stop them rather than teach children how to use words to resolve the conflict.

As parents, we have to become obsessed with observing kindness to become successful at encouraging it. Doing so also changes us. When we begin to notice the generous, empathetic actions of children, we get a more balanced picture. It's easy to characterize negative moments as happening more often than they actually do. When we get good at catching positive actions, we also realize that we can trick children into being kind even when they are feeling selfish and grumpy.

In Faber and Mazlish's first book, *Liberated Parents, Liberated Children,* one of the mothers realizes that her daughter has become disturbingly self-centered. In an effort to apply positive reinforcement, she tries to find a time when the girl demonstrates kindness, but to no avail. Finally, one day, after the girl has almost finished eating a whole box of cookies, the mother slyly takes the cookie box and thanks the girl for saving some for her brothers. The girl looks at her mother in disbelief. She had no altruistic intention of saving any cookies, but she goes along with it. Her mother's appreciation for her "kindness" has an impact. At first, the girl doesn't see herself as a thoughtful person, but her mother's repeated attempts succeed in undoing negative and unsociable behavior.

This miraculous process reminds me of a quote by Johann von Goethe: "Treat people as if they were what they ought to be, and you

help them to become what they are capable of being." It's easy to promote a child's laziness or lack of generosity. If we merely berate them
repeatedly for not wanting to do chores or for taking the last cookie,
they will identify with being lazy and selfish. But if we can train ourselves to watch and acknowledge positive moments, no matter how
brief, we discover that we have the power to help children grow into
the thoughtful and kind people they are capable of being. The goal of
bringing out their best qualities lies at the heart of all effective discipline and good parenting.

**Rate yourself on observing and appreciating positive
actions, on a scale of 1 to 10.**

CHAPTER 5

Discipline by Design, Not Default

Find Somebody to Watch

Example is not the main thing in influencing others. It
is the only thing.

ALBERT SCHWEITZER

Emma got in such intense power struggles with her two-year-old son
Billy that he would sometimes hurt her. He was big for his age, and
when he got mad he would hit her or kick her. Sometimes he threw
things at her, and it scared her. But she had no idea how to take
charge. "My parents were both really permissive, and I didn't have
good role models for setting limits. I tried to do what parenting books
advised, but that isn't the same as seeing someone relate to a child
well. I could hear that my voice didn't communicate any authority.
That's why Billy didn't listen. If I tried to stop him physically, he would
fight me. I have strong values about parenting, and I didn't want to be
yelling or hitting him. But I didn't want to be his victim either."

In Emma's case, it was especially important for her to take charge
with Billy because she suffers from lupus. Restraining him physically
proved painful for her. Lupus also restricts her from staying in the sun-
light, and she felt it was imperative that Billy listen to her about getting in the car quickly.

One night Emma met Phyllis, a speaker at her parents' group. As
Phyllis spoke, Emma realized that Phyllis embodied all her highest
ideals about being a parent, and she wanted to learn from her. Emma
asked if they could talk sometime and got Phyllis's number. Phyllis
invited Emma to take her positive parenting class.

Emma and her husband count the decision to accept that invitation as the turning point in their relationship with Billy. The techniques they learned stopped the power struggles they were having with their preschooler. In addition, the two women became friends, and Emma had opportunities to watch Phyllis with her children. "Watching the ways she related to them was so valuable for me. I could see that my hard work would pay off. I listened to the tone of voice she used when she offered choices or followed up on a request. I loved the ways she related to her children. Whenever I was in a difficult situation, I would ask myself what Phyllis would do, and she was always happy for me to call."

Emma's way of handling Billy gradually became more authoritative—the kind of relating she had never had a model for, when she was growing up. Today he is six, and she reports proudly that they almost never have power struggles. His teachers say his behavior is excellent. "He could have been a difficult child because he has such high energy, but I've learned how to work with him."

We aren't taught to look for role models when we become parents. Perhaps that's because our society doesn't acknowledge people who are gifted at relating to children. We have mentors in academic pursuits and in careers, so why not look for positive examples in the most important endeavor we will ever undertake—becoming the mother or father we want to be? All we have to do is look for someone who possesses the qualities we want to learn, and then watch what they do. As one mother said, "No one knows how to handle every parenting situation flawlessly, but some people know how to handle some situations better than others."

Most parents have a vague image of the parent they would like to become, though the specific behaviors they want to acquire may be fuzzy. If we take the time to observe what's actually happening when people work with children successfully, we will notice their tone of voice, their body language, and the words they use. The concrete things people do can help us bring our ideals into reality.

Sometimes we might choose a psychotherapist as our role model. If we don't want to repeat the way our parents reacted when we expressed our feelings, we can watch the way our therapist responds to us. This type of role modeling provides an even deeper effect because the therapist teaches us to reparent ourselves. When we learn to function better internally, it is much easier to interact well with our children.

Whether we try to emulate an acquaintance or a professional, remembering the old adage "Seeing is believing" helps us see the skills we want to learn, as others put them into action. We get to observe what the process of offering limited choices or implementing logical consequences actually looks like.

List five people whose relationships with children you admire. Next to each name, record the qualities or skills you've observed in them.

Give Them a Choice

> If I were to say to a child, "Ball playing in the house bothers me; you can play with it outside or put it away. You decide." I had better be prepared to take the ball away if he continues. I could say as I remove the ball, "Jimmy, I see you decided."
>
> **HAIM GINOTT**

A man standing in the bank parking lot explains to his little girl that they need to get in their car now. She begins to scream and pulls on his hand. I watch, wondering whether he will become impatient at her sudden "irrational" response. In an effort to deal with public situations quickly, it's easy for parents to lose composure. In this situation, however, the father responds matter-of-factly, "I see you don't want to get in the car, but we have to go now. Do you want me to hold your hand, or should I carry you?" He had already started to pick her up as I walked past, leaving me impressed by his calm detachment.

By offering clear choices, this parent kept an awkward little situation from escalating into a distressing big one. He demonstrated an important discipline skill—one that I can break down best by stating what he didn't do.

He didn't launch into a lengthy explanation about why they had to leave, to pressure his daughter into his point of view.

Nor did he undermine his own authority by repeating the choice over and over, or offering a variety of choices, waiting for her to comply.

He didn't try to bribe her.

Nor did he hurt her feelings by saying, "You know we have to go, what are you crying about? You're being a baby, and you're going to make us late."

By giving her the power to decide how she wanted to get in the car, and following through quickly, this parent showed that providing children with limited options can prevent prolonged upset at the moment, or even prevent a pattern of conflict in the long run. I could picture the little girl in her car seat already happily chattering to her dad feeling that she has some power over her life.

Like anyone pressured to do what someone else wants, children resist our uncompromising efforts to get them to obey. To their own detriment, they also learn to tune us out. Offering clear-cut choices provides them an increment of power and the warning of what will happen next. Following through calmly communicates that we mean business.

But sometimes the choices that we could offer aren't obvious, particularly with irksome situations that recur. Because of this, it helps to think creatively, ahead of time, about what options we want to offer.

My children wouldn't listen to me, even though I asked them many times to stop verbally dueling and jabbing at each other physically while I was driving. Explaining the dangers didn't impress them, which made me feel even crazier. Finally I thought of the choice I could offer, and the first time I tried it, I wondered if it would work. I pulled the car over to the side of the road and said, "You have a choice. Either you can ride in silence without touching each other, or we can sit here by the side of the road." Then I pulled out a book or magazine and read while they decided what they wanted to do. It took a few times of stopping the car before they started saying, "We know, Mom; it's time for silence." You can imagine my satisfaction. Later I wrote an article on how much we came to enjoy those "sips of silence."

Having the freedom to choose between one action and another is one of the great gifts of life. The more we make conscious choices, rather than acting without thinking, the more power we feel to steer our course. We help children to learn to be aware that they can make good decisions when we offer choices clearly and show that we respect what they choose. Offering choices respectfully provides the basis of teaching children through logical consequences.

Record some situations with your child that trigger your frustration, and list what choices you could offer him or her.

Let the Consequence Do the Talking

If you would persuade, you must appeal to interest rather than intellect.

BENJAMIN FRANKLIN

Barbara talked to her two elementary-aged children repeatedly about getting ready to leave on time in the morning. As a teacher in the same school that they attended, she had to be in her room before her students started arriving. But Adam and Leila had no interest in getting to school early, and tended to dawdle. Their mother finally warned them that their slow pace would result in a consequence: "If you can't get ready on time tomorrow, you'll have to get dressed in the car."

Her words made no impression—at least not right away. The next morning, Adam and Leila were still fooling around when it came time to leave. Without getting angry, Barbara carried their clothes and a blanket to the car and drove away. After circling the block, she found her two children in their pajamas on the porch. "Mom, what are you doing?" they yelled. While she drove to school, the children, much to their chagrin, had to get dressed under the blanket to protect their privacy.

The next time Barbara took their things to the car, they knew she meant it. But they had to get dressed in the car two or three more times before they learned to meet her deadline. In the end, it was their own interest that persuaded them. They wanted to get dressed in the privacy of their home. The intellectual argument that they should get ready to prevent their mother from arriving late had no effect on them, while the consequence left a lasting impression.

In *Children: The Challenge*, probably the bestselling book on child discipline ever written, Rudolf Dreikurs says, "Natural consequences represent the pressures of reality . . . they are always efficient." The key, he says, is using a positive tone when warning children about the repercussions of their actions. Barbara's attitude was amiable every time she brought her children's clothes to the car. Had her tone been chastising, it would have cast the consequence as a punishment, which would probably have bred resentment.

Recently, a loving father told me about a fight he had with his four-year-old son one morning. The boy had disobeyed him by eating candy. The father threw the candy in the garbage, saying sternly, "That's your consequence."

Later when they had to leave the house, the father couldn't find his car keys. His son said, "I hid them; that's your consequence."

Employing a cheerful attitude while we allow the consequences of negative behavior to occur preserves our harmonious relationships with children. It also prevents arguing. Think of these consequences as a force all their own—like gravity. What goes up must come down. We're not punishing, we're allowing nature to run its course. We can even express sympathy for the child: "I'm sorry you can't watch TV, but you didn't do your homework on time the way we discussed."

Keep in mind, though, that once we warn the child of the consequences, we don't need to talk about them much or go out of our way to explain the impetus behind them. Children will quickly adapt to suit their own interests. The consequence does most of the work. One father liked the fact that the instructor in his parent education class compared consequences to a free golf swing. The instructor's analogy made sense: "If you relax and allow the natural force of gravity to move the club, the whole swing is easier and more effective. It's that way with consequences. They do the job for you."

As with Barbara's decision to stop lecturing and take off for school on time, the best consequences motivate children to do better next time and allow us to set the boundaries we need to function well.

> **Think back to your childhood and how adults tried to teach you to behave differently. How did you feel when your parents used a forceful or critical tone of voice when correcting you? Did your parents set boundaries that helped you to respect their needs? Can you remember a consequence that taught you a lesson?**

Stand by Your Boundaries

A boundary is a "property line" that defines where one person ends and someone else begins.

DR. HENRY CLOUD AND DR. JOHN TOWNSEND

At lunchtime recess, five-year-old Bryan sobs on the school playground, pulling on the sleeve of his mother's blouse. Other children look on with anxious curiosity. "I want to go with you," Bryan cries. Caryl has left her job early to pick up Bryan's twin sister Regina, who has spiked a fever. I watch as Caryl kneels down, communicating with Bryan in a soft, steady voice. "I'm not going to take you with me because Regina is sick, and I have to give her my full attention. I also have to talk to the doctor, and I can't do it with the two of you acting silly."

"It's not fair," Bryan shrieks. "I want to be with you. I won't act silly, I promise!" Caryl stands up to signal her departure. Her demeanor is firm but not unsympathetic. "I know you want to come, and I wish you could, Bryan. But I can only handle taking one child to the doctor today. I'll spend time with you after we get back."

I realize, then, that in this little exchange, I am watching a remarkable process. Caryl is not only allowing Bryan to express his anger, she is validating his right to have fiery feelings and her right to stand by her boundaries.

In other, less emotionally attuned generations, "normal" parental behavior might have included shaming Bryan for "crying like a baby in front of other people," slapping him for not accepting "no," and maybe even threatening not to pick him up at all if he continued with this "embarrassing scene." Before parents were aware of the lifelong consequences of shaming and of threats of abandonment, extinguishing a child's anger felt like a parental duty—the only way to maintain authority.

I can understand that. It's taken me years to sense that the unempathetic, uncompromising anger of a kid can trigger me into reacting like a hurt child who wants to defend herself. Many conflicts between adults and children turn into a standoff between two emotionally overwhelmed five year olds, or else an adult caves in, but with resentment.

But Caryl is doing things differently, and she has demonstrated her awareness of a basic principle of mental health. She knows where Bryan's feelings end and her own begin.

In his book *The Family*, John Bradshaw describes a mature person as having "marked ego boundaries." I can observe that Caryl's assertion of a boundary helps her protect her good mood. Her unspoken stance—I can understand you're upset, but I'm not letting it change my mood or my actions—helps Bryan gain awareness of his separate sense of self. Seconds after she leaves, he runs off to play with his friends, no doubt relieved that he can't overwhelm his mother with his own confusing feelings.

Like so many parents, Caryl is learning that setting firm boundaries enables her to protect her emotional and physical well-being and allows her to function optimally as a parent. But I know that this learning process is extremely difficult and often accompanied by feelings of guilt and confusion.

Had Caryl's boundary collapsed under Bryan's tidal wave of emotional pressure, an unpleasant time at the doctor's office might have sabotaged her calm and changed the rest of their day. But Caryl's ability to "stay adult" in the face of Bryan's anger has meaning far beyond the preservation of one afternoon. One of the best things parents can do is set a boundary that helps them hold on to their good mood even while they acknowledge a child's upset feelings. Whenever we are able to put an ideal into action, we pave the way to doing it again, and to demonstrating to others that it can be done.

Stop and think about what boundaries you set to maintain your emotional and physical balance.
Record an incident when you were able to allow a child her own feelings, without letting them affect yours.

CHAPTER 6

See the Opportunity in the Obstacle

Tolerate Indecision

What confused me . . . was how much freedom I was supposed to give Sam. I'm unclear about the fine line between good parenting and being overprotective. I get stumped by the easy test questions like whether I should let Sam ride his two wheeler for several blocks without me, when I secretly want to run alongside him like a golden retriever.

ANNE LAMOTT

Would you let your child paraglide with a trained instructor for his seventh birthday, if he desperately wanted to? That's the real-life quandary author Anne Lamott details in her book *Traveling Mercies: Some Thoughts on Faith*. At a writer's conference in Idaho, Anne meets a paragliding instructor who turns to her son Sam, inviting him to go for a birthday ride two days later. Ann says she wants to ponder the decision, and the instructor says he can tentatively hold the date. As Sam begs her to go, half of her thinks she owes him this birthday present, since he is a thousand miles from home and can't celebrate turning seven with his friends. The other half knows it would be insane to allow her child to jump off a mountain. But her indecision allows her to process the answer in a most interesting way.

She calls some friends to ask their opinion. Half think she should let Sam go, and the other half consider the stunt ridiculously dangerous. That night at dinner she asks a couple what they think. The man favors Sam's side, and the woman insists he is far too young. As the couple's argument gets more heated, Ann's indecision mounts.

Music starts playing, and she gets up to dance by herself. As she moves to the music, she remembers a simple but powerful technique for decision making, once offered to her by a priest. She gets very quiet internally and asks herself how she would feel if Sam went. Her heart immediately leaps into her throat. Then she thinks about saying no to Sam, and her body feels euphoric. Thinking can take us only so far; her body knows the answer. Realizing her true feelings, Ann phones and cancels the paragliding date. Later she is surprised when Sam is a good sport about it.

How do we make decisions about our children when there is no clear-cut, right answer? Conventional wisdom would have us believe indecision is a weakness and we should be clear about what we believe. The beauty of Anne Lamott's story is the tolerance she demonstrates for her own confusion, even as she pokes fun at it. She doesn't cave in to Sam's pressure. She stays with her discomfort until she discovers her real feelings and decides, this time, to honor them. She can't handle her son paragliding at the age of seven. He will have to wait until he is older to soar "like an eagle."

It seems to me that indecision is often the only sane response to all of the crazy decisions a parent has to make. Is it safe for them to walk to the store or ride their bikes around the block? Should we let our children see the movie all the other kids are going to? What about the all-night party after the dance?

Our indecision signals us that we can't give our children an instant answer, no matter how much they plead. Sometimes we need more information or the chance to tune in to our children more effectively. Perhaps we want to confer with other parents or gather courage to stand by our convictions. Other times we have to be quiet and tune in to our bodies before we know what we are really feeling and why. Then we can ask if we want to work through our feelings or go with them.

There is no one right way to handle decisions about our kids. But one of the best things parents can do is to be honest about their confusion with themselves and others. Doing so honors our commitment to discovering our highest truth and living it. Sometimes confusion just provides the internal space to ask questions of ourselves and get clear on our priorities.

Think of some decisions you've made that honor what's important to you as a parent or someone who cares for a child. List those decisions in terms of priority.

Reward with Time

The butterfly counts not months but moments, and has
time enough.

RABINDRANATH TAGORE

Few parents haven't been stressed by morning or evening routines—trying to get kids out of bed and out the door, making sure that evening baths, homework, and bedtime happen in a timely manner. Under pressure, it's easy to forget that kids aren't as motivated as we are to rush out the door so we won't be late to work, or to cut evenings short to jump into bed. I've discovered that one of the secrets of changing these routines is to give children something that lifts their mood and motivates them to cooperate.

Of the hundreds of parents I've consulted with about making mornings and evenings more enjoyable, I love Diane and her daughter Erin's story the best. Erin hated saying goodbye before preschool. She would scream so loudly her mother could hear her in the school as she drove away. This behavior went on for a period of about eight months. She had fun once she settled down, but the teachers worried about why her morning upset was so intense.

When I met with Diane about Erin's distress, I learned that not only was Diane a devoted parent to a preschooler and a baby but also the CEO of her own company. We talked about the behaviors that sour a parent's mood in the morning: a child refusing to leave the TV and get dressed and then arguing about what to wear. Quickly, the reasons for Erin's behaviors seemed clear to me. I have seen over and over that a child's morning goodbye reflects the feelings that have gone on between parent and child that morning. No wonder Erin cried in the mornings; she and Diane had argued from the time they got up.

I proposed a solution that I have observed to work successfully on countless occasions. I advised Diane to reward Erin with fifteen or twenty minutes of having fun as a perk for getting ready on time. Erin would have an incentive to get ready on time, and her mood would improve after having time with her mom. I told Diane this secret worked equally well in the evenings and that no video game, TV program, or toy could compare with the reward of spending time with her.

Diane's expression revealed her incredulity. "How can I possibly spend time with Erin playing when I can barely get myself and the baby ready? I'm always running late." We talked more about the impossibility of mornings, and then she had to leave. However, after a couple of months Erin suddenly changed. She entered the schoolroom skipping in the morning and smiled at the teachers. She said goodbye to her mother easily. Her teachers were stunned by the dramatic turnaround. Finally, after two weeks of Erin's bright smile, I asked Diane about Erin's mood change.

Diane's look softened and I thought she might cry. "I started spending time with Erin in the mornings," she said. "And I got my girl back. I started getting up a little earlier so I could be with her. It's a wonderful way to start the day." I was touched by the effort Diane was making and the dramatic difference it made in Erin's day.

It's hard to understand what a powerful motivator rewarding our children with time can be. Over the years I have observed that planning regular playtime is one of best things parents can do. It positively affects almost every ongoing conflict between parents and kids. To understand it, I ask parents to fantasize about their own lives. Imagine that your partner or a friend surprised you by bringing you flowers and saying, "I've been missing you so much, I need time with you. Is there anything you want to do?" How would you describe the change in your mood? Suddenly, we want to do things for the other person; we feel open and cooperative. That's the way our children feel, too.

Understanding her daughter's needs helped Diane to make her daughter's well-being the top priority. As the adult, she took responsibility for restoring their closeness.

> **Keep track of how often you and your child have special alone time together having fun. Consistency sends the message that time together means just as much to you as it does to your child.**

I'm the Adult

> I longed for my mother to be more adult when I was a
> child, though I couldn't have told you at the time what
> that meant. Thinking back, I wish she could have given
> me the sense that she could handle whatever came her
> way, even when life was hard.
>
> **ANONYMOUS**

Jackie says her life is coming unglued. Things are tense at her insurance company because of the economy, and her husband has been out of work for months. Meanwhile, her mother is visiting with the hope of finding a place nearby. She asks every day how David's job search is going, and it takes all Jackie's self-control not to boil over and say, "The same as it was yesterday." Her nine-year-old daughter, Megan, also keeps asking if Jackie's okay.

Jackie has decided to talk to her daughter about being stressed. She assures me, however, that she has no intention of making a plea for more consideration and support. Actually, she wants to convince Megan that no matter how challenging life appears right now, she needn't worry about her mom. Jackie wants Megan's childhood to be free from the anxiety that she felt about her mother when she was a child. "I've gone through years of therapy to understand my own dynamics with my mom, and I don't want to repeat them. I want Megan to feel lighthearted and have fun. I know from experience that if I don't talk about what's going on, she's going to be convinced that she is the problem." Jackie knows that Megan can't help but pick up on her feelings, even if she doesn't say anything.

Biologically our children are tuned to our inner state. In an eloquent synthesis of neurobiology and psychology entitled *A General Theory of Love*, Drs. Thomas Lewis, Fari Amini, and Richard Lannon describe how a "primordial area of the brain, far older than reasoning or thinking" propels us to be affected by each other's unspoken emotions. The ways brains link with one another are part of the story of human survival. The infant has to learn to read the subtle signals of the caretaker's inner state in order to feel the security of attachment.

Jackie knows that her daughter's ability to pick up her upsets is normal. But she feels that her counseling has allowed her to sense her daughter's desire to fix things. What separates Jackie's perceptions from those of parents who have not reflected on these issues is that her priority is to stay "adult" and make her daughter feel secure. "I'm going to tell her that everybody has difficult feelings sometimes. When I have those feelings, I may need to be alone for a little while, but she doesn't have to worry about me. I know how to take care of myself."

It's actually helpful for a nine year old to hear that her mother can be stressed, frustrated, or sad and may need time alone to process her feelings. One of the best things parents can do is answer their children reassuringly when they ask, "Are you okay?" A person can say, "I'm tired from a full day at work, but I'll be fine after a cup of tea." Parents need to find opportunities to show that they can handle adversity, and to let their children know that they don't have to worry about them. When parents talk about the tools they use for managing stress, kids learn that intense feelings can be managed and obstacles overcome.

Jackie can be proud of all the work she has done to learn what being an adult really means. It's easy when we're overwhelmed by life's circumstances to forget that our moods are affecting our children. Jackie is fortunate to be a mother now, when people are conscious that taking on their parents' emotional burdens keeps children from putting energy into their own development. Nature has programmed them to be aware of our distress, but showing them we can handle stress and telling them they are not at fault are among the best things a parent can do. Reassuring Megan that her mother can handle what life offers her helps Jackie to acknowledge her own hard-earned strength and to remember to be grateful for her own growth.

Picture a time when your mother or father's life seemed overly stressful. How did they handle your concerns? What reassurances would you have liked from them?

I Am Grateful

Gratitude unlocks the fullness of life. It turns what we have into enough, and more.

MELODY BEATTIE

When Georgia's son Ted broke his leg, last year, the staff kept her out of the emergency room because she might "freak out" and make things worse for him. Since she wasn't crying and she was communicating calmly, Georgia didn't understand. But the doctor was harsh and said he had to set Ted's leg without any sedation since he had just eaten lunch, and it was going to be very painful. Georgia paced the hall, listening to her son shriek for what seemed like hours. Yet even though she wanted to be with him, from the beginning Georgia was aware of a deep sense of gratitude. "When I got to Children's Hospital I was hit with a huge realization. My son will leave this hospital and get better, but many children here will never go home again. That instantly put my life in perspective and [I realized] how lucky I was that nothing worse had happened. I began to say thank you—thank you for the break happening at school where there was immediate help, thank you that I could be reached on the phone, thank you for the kind people in the school office and in the ambulance. I couldn't stop saying thank you."

Georgia remembers the professor in a psychology course saying that in the *I Ching*, the Chinese book of divination, there is one symbol that means both crisis and opportunity. Looking back to that day at the hospital, she sees how much learning both she and Ted have done.

Georgia says the wave of gratitude that swept over her also helped her son, when she communicated it to him. He could have been angry at the boy who tripped and fell on top of him, causing the break. Instead, the first thing he wanted to do the same day his leg was set was to write to that boy and tell him not to worry. "He developed a feeling for people in pain. He doesn't just sympathize; he really empathizes now because he has been there and knows what it's like. He also understands people in wheelchairs or using walkers because he had to do that for two months. Can you imagine how antsy an eight year old would get watching everyone else jump around and play sports? I had to volunteer in the school office for two months because he couldn't go to the bathroom by himself and didn't want anyone else to take him."

Think how different Georgia's experience would have been if she hadn't cultivated an attitude of gratitude with her son. There could have been lingering anger at the doctor who kept her out of the ER, not to mention anger at life for putting her son through such suffering. For Georgia, gratitude was a blessing that kept her focused on the positive parts of the experience.

It's easy to be grateful when none of our loved ones are sick or in pain, when we have a job, a good relationship, and a child who is doing well in school. It's harder to say thank you when things aren't going the way we want. As the saying goes, "Want to make God laugh? Just tell Him your plans!"

What is the wisdom inherent in offering up our thankfulness instead of our rage when apparent misfortune besets us or our dear ones?

Our attitude of gratitude helps the people around us, especially our children, who look to us as role models. It also heals us. When we see our problems as opportunities for growth and adopt a grateful attitude toward them, we program our subconscious minds to let go of fear, concentrate on the positive, and surround us with a feeling of blessing. When we teach our children to look for reasons to be thankful, we do our part to create a new generation that is more conscious of their ability to choose positive emotions. We can also offer thanks that we live in an age when the world offers us the tools and knowledge we need to bolster our children's growth.

Make a list of the top ten things in your life that you are grateful for.

Think Like an Expert

Somewhere, something incredible is waiting to be
known.

ANONYMOUS

When I met Terry and Eric, their two-year-old daughter, Marissa, had
just started to backslide in her verbal development. At fourteen
months, she had spoken with an amazing two-hundred-word vocabu-
lary. Afterwards, she had her measles, mumps, and rubella vaccina-
tion, ran a high fever, and stayed in the hospital for two weeks. Then,
she started losing her speech, finally grunting to ask for what she
wanted. Terry didn't buy into prognoses that her daughter was autis-
tic. She had heard stories of similar cases connected to the binding
agent in the MMR vaccinations when they are administered together.
She found links on the Internet to studies corroborating what she had
heard about the MMR and learned that giving the vaccinations together is banned in Japan. Terry and Eric consulted with many professionals and read everything they could on Marissa's problem.

Terry decided to follow the advice of a teacher at Marissa's new
special education preschool. The teacher suggested talking to Marissa
continually as if she were still normal. Terry left her job to stay home
with her daughter, and she talked to her constantly, in spite of the lack
of response. Over time, Marissa's speech started to improve as the
result of speech therapy at school and talking at home. By the time
Marissa was five, Terry and Eric were faced with an unexpected decision. Should they put her in normal kindergarten even though her

speech was still difficult to understand? They were working with a number of professionals, but ultimately the decision was up to them. Terry said it required a huge leap of faith, but finally they had to trust their intuition. They enrolled Marissa in a kindergarten that encourages parent participation, and Terry volunteered in the class every day to help other children understand Marissa's speech.

Now in her "normal" third grade, few people would guess that Marissa was once deemed as a candidate for special education. She scores high academically, and her speech is almost completely normal. Interestingly, she talks now about the things her parents told her when no one knew if she understood. Recently she remembered a white balloon that had escaped from her hand and Terry's explanations about it flying away. Terry and Eric are touched by Marissa's memories and gratified that they chose to follow the right professional's advice and their own intuition about helping their daughter.

We live in a time when we feel empowered to become knowledgeable advocates for our children's mental and physical health. If we make the leap to thinking like an expert, we can learn much of what's known about a subject. That means sifting through lots of information and consulting with other people who have expertise, then making our hypotheses about the most effective course. Looking for our own answers in the same way an expert would is one of the best things we can do.

Terry and Eric's story reminds me of the miraculous efforts of two other parents, Mikaela and Augusto Odone. Neither was a scientist, but they found a way to arrest their son's terminal disease. Their story of searching for answers in scientific studies and bravely coming up with their own conclusions, ultimately saving their son's life, is told in the 1992 movie *Lorenzo's Oil*. Today the world is full of countless tales of parents pursuing the knowledge they need and trusting their instincts. They aren't usually extraordinary life-or-death stories, or even as dramatic as speaking versus being mute, but they celebrate our ability to develop child-rearing expertise.

As Alvin Toffler, author of *Future Shock*, wrote, "Knowledge is knowing—or knowing where to find out."

Developing resources provides us with the ability to make more informed decisions, but we have to remember that our most profound knowing often comes from our own intuitions and perceptions.

Look up a child-related issue online, or talk to a friend about what she has learned about an issue. Keep files on all the resources that come out of your exploration.
Which studies corroborate your feelings about the subject?

CHAPTER 7

Know Them by Heart

Stop the World to Really Listen

It's helpful to pay attention to the quality of our attention and to practice the art of pure listening—so that you can give this gift to children at least some of the time.

HARRIET LERNER

One evening I arrived punctually for an appointment at an editor's house to discuss a manuscript. "I'll be a few minutes," she said. "I'm having a conversation with my daughter." I sat down on the couch in the living room, where I could see her at the dining room table with an adorable blond girl about eleven years old. As soon as she sat down again, they started talking. Actually, the girl spoke in a hesitant way, and the mother leaned forward and listened. But it was the kind of listening people don't witness every day.

I was struck by the expression on the mother's face as she concentrated her full attention on what her daughter was saying. I could see that she was checking in visually on her daughter's feelings as she talked. If I could have interpreted her nonverbal cues, they would have said, "You can tell me anything, and I will still love you just as much. There is nothing more important to me than hearing what you have to say."

One of the things I have learned from my observations is that listening to kids almost always involves stopping what you are doing at the most inconvenient times. A colleague is waiting. The dinner needs cooking, or we simply have to be somewhere in a hurry. I know at least one parent who pulled her car to the side of the road to offer her full attention while her child discussed an important school problem, and she sat there until he finished. Of course, she didn't do this every time she picked him up. But stopping the car even once demonstrated her willingness to listen.

When I'm in a classroom, I am often faced with interruptions—a spill that needs mopping, a phone call, or an adult who has a matter to discuss. Any of these events can make me forget the children in front of me. Since the world will constantly present distractions, I have to stay on the lookout not to lose my focus. I have to show the children that I am there to concentrate on them.

The importance of giving full attention came home to me a few years ago when I saw Dr. John Gottman's film *The Heart of Parenting*. I was mesmerized by the clips of parents stopping to check on their children's feelings. The film talks about his research at the University of Washington, which shows that having their feelings noticed and validated reduces stress hormones in a child's bloodstream. As I watched *The Heart of Parenting*, I realized that I was watching a new art form, not in film, but in parent/child relationships.

I felt the same way when I questioned a young mother in New York about the wonderful way she related to her two young children while I was visiting.

"How did you learn to give your children such complete attention when you talk to them?" I asked. Her answer surprised me.

"I read a book on how to love them," she said frankly. "Why not? All the magazines tell you now to create romance and make a man feel loved. So I worked on learning to show my children how much I appreciate them."

How do parents remember to stop and focus on a child in an age that pulls them in so many directions at once?

It helps to remember that we can only make a difference in a child's life by joining her fully in the present moment. We actually have the capacity to nourish a child's belief that she is worthy of being heard. If we do stop everything to listen, she will be more likely to listen to herself and develop confidence in her own best knowing.

> **Try role-playing with your spouse or a friend. Listen with total attention (no questions or interruptions) as your partner speaks for five minutes about any subject she chooses. Then switch places so you can speak.**

Analyze the Effect of Activities

We worry about what a child will be tomorrow. Yet, we forget he is someone today.

STACIA TAUSCHER

I was surprised when Phillip's mother, Carol, told me he was balking about going to first grade. In preschool, he stood out as bright and interested in everything. Now he was crying about school each morning, and the teachers said he didn't pay attention. Carol noticed that he seemed unable to concentrate on his new soccer team, too. At home, he was grouchy. One day he threw such an explosive tantrum that Carol told him he couldn't watch TV or play video games for three weeks. Afterwards, she thought her reaction was extreme but decided to uphold it. Concerned that he was actually overtired, she also took him off the soccer team and restricted his play dates to weekends. She had signed him up because his friends were on the team and she didn't want him to get behind in sports. She also began putting him to bed an hour earlier.

After a week, these changes brought dramatic results. Suddenly Phillip liked school, and his teachers said his concentration was good and he finished his work right on time. He seemed more peaceful at home and spent time climbing trees in the backyard. Carol began to see that Phillip was flourishing as she reduced the amount of stimulation in his life. Now with the three-week hiatus from TV and video games coming to an end, her plan is to restrict these activities to two hours a week. There have been so many benefits from cutting out those activities, and she wants him to continue exploring the outdoors.

Phillip didn't know he was tired from trying to learn how to read and memorize the rules of soccer at the same time. Nor did he know he needed more restful activities than the stimulation of TV and video games. Yet, cutting down on activity restored his balance. Extra activities weren't what he needed during this crucial year of learning.

On the other hand, at another stage of development, dedication to a physical activity may actually help a child handle life's stresses. Sheila told me that her teenage daughter Megan's immersion in ballet, even taking classes five to six times a week, helped her to throw off adolescent confusion and turmoil. "She never wanted to be a ballerina. But she loved taking classes, and when she came home from ballet, it was as if she had shed the troubles of the day." When Megan was in elementary school, many of her friends attended a variety of extracurricular activities. Sheila knew that more activity wasn't necessarily better. She encouraged Megan to devote herself to one activity that she loved. Megan's development has been helped by ballet because she has enjoyed the process of dancing without thinking about where it would lead.

I admire parents like Carol and Sheila who look at the effects of activities on their children's lives in the present, instead of thinking of extracurricular activities as important so children can compete with others in the future. Children don't have the sophistication or judgment to say, "This refreshes me," or "I'm too overscheduled." One of the best things we can do is analyze what activities keep our children's lives in balance and enjoyable right now. Watching them helps us to stay in touch with what they need as they mature and learn to make those decisions for themselves.

Did your parents decide on your activities when you were a child, or did they listen to your feelings? Did you tend to be overstructured or need more to do?

Tune Them In to Their Inner Voices

The outside world works hard to make a child deaf to
his own warning bell.

ADELE FABER AND ELAINE MAZLISH

From the time Allie was in preschool, she and her mother, Karen,
always stopped to look at animals, especially dogs. Seeing a dog at the
park, they would stand back and talk about what they thought the
furry creature was like. What kind of dog was he? What mood was he
in? After observing for a while, they asked themselves the most important question of all: "What does each of us feel? Is this is a friendly
dog, or does he look dangerous?"

Karen says she wanted to teach her daughter to pause and tune in to
what her inner voice said about engaging with an animal. "We both liked
playing the game of accessing our feelings about a dog and sharing what
we noticed. It was a nonthreatening way to talk about dangers." Now
that Allie is seven, Karen has a new focus for their observations: making the bridge from animals to people. She wants Allie to pay attention
to her feelings about people—other kids and grownups. As one part of
that process, they took a workshop about how to avoid threats such as
kidnapping or molestation. The class taught them how to sense potential danger by remaining alert.

Recently, two men in a car pulled up in front of Karen's house and
asked for directions, while the mother and daughter were outside.
Once they departed, Karen asked Allie if she noticed the space she
had kept between herself and the car, to maintain a safety zone. They

also discussed their impressions of the two men. This kind of personal analysis has much more meaning for a child than simply saying, "Don't talk to strangers."

Their discussions, however, have not been limited to potential threats. They also talk about dealing with people in other situations. A neighbor started yelling at Karen a while back. Karen was confused but said, "I'm sorry I made you so angry."

The neighbor shouted, "I'm not angry."

When they got in the car, seven-year-old Allie commented, "Olivia isn't good at noticing her own feelings, is she?"

Teaching a child to pay attention to others and to her own feelings is one of the best things we can do. The process allows a child to begin assessing situations for herself. It may take more time, but it's worth it. Recently, on a snow trip, Allie said she didn't want to take a ski lesson, even though the other children on the trip were delighted to try the new activity. It's easy for parents to want to pressure a child to overcome her hesitancy, thinking they know better and the child will have fun. But Allie's parents want her to feel that tuning in to her inner voice is the foundation for making good decisions now and in the future.

Karen invited Allie to go tubing in the snow. Allie wanted to walk over and observe the activity before committing herself. Once she saw the tubes, she agreed. Allowing Allie to check in with her feelings took about an hour longer, but Karen says the extra time allowed her daughter to approach the activity with more confidence.

In his groundbreaking book *Emotional Intelligence*, Daniel Goleman describes this intuitive process as an exercise in noticing the reactions of others, being aware of our feelings about them, and learning to interact with others skillfully. Observing others involves valuing the process of pausing and looking before rushing into a situation. Allie has become an emotionally intelligent seven year old.

Talking about what feelings "tell" them about various situations has been a jumping-off point for further conversations between mother and daughter. Karen has been able to keep track of the changes in Allie's life and in her internal being. Now that Allie is seven, they have a closeness that allows them to talk more and more.

Even with trust, however, children won't always share their feelings and concerns. Sometimes emotions feel too overwhelming, or a sense of shame accompanies them. As children grow older and form close relationships with peers, talking to parents about friends may seem like a betrayal. That's when parents need to learn how to assess their children's well-being in new ways, like reading between the lines of their verbal and nonverbal communication.

Imagine your child in a challenging situation when you aren't there. How do you want her inner voice and her connection with her feelings to help her? What preparation can you give to strengthen her inner resources?

Read Between the Lines

The best thing to read when trying to raise a child is the child.

SUSAN ISAACS AND MARTI KELLER

The first sign that something was wrong in Katie's world arose as a medical issue. Though she had no history of asthma, the nine year old started telling her parents she couldn't breathe. Her mother, Abbe, suspected Katie was having panic attacks, but her daughter told her there was nothing wrong. Their doctor also thought the problem was anxiety and asked Katie how her friendships were going. Katie again responded that things were okay, but the way she looked down when she answered made Abbe want to find out more.

On a class field trip, Abbe observed that something had gone very wrong in her daughter's relationships. Katie's close friends didn't speak to her on the outing, and one girl tried to push her during a group activity. Dismayed, Abbe asked Katie why her friends had seemed so unfriendly. Katie sadly admitted that they had refused to play with her for weeks. She had no idea why. They called her names if she tried to join them. Abbe didn't know what to do; Katie had been friends with these girls for years. She told Katie she understood how sad she must be feeling. Abbe's own sadness was overwhelming, and her husband was furious. Abbe looked for ways to help them through this trying time.

Soon afterwards, she saw Rachel Simmons, the author of *Odd Girl Out: The Hidden Culture of Aggression in Girls* on *The Oprah*

Winfrey Show. In her extensive research, Simmons found that anger and jealousy between the closest friends often resulted in a girl being suddenly rejected and bombarded with mean notes and insults. Since the girls appeared well behaved, teachers were usually unaware of their behavior.

After hearing about bullying, Abbe's angry impulse was to call the girls' parents. However, after speaking to a counselor specializing in children's social relationships, she decided against it. Instead, on the therapist's advice, she helped Katie to think of comebacks to the girls' taunts to give her confidence.

Abbe also talked to the school staff. As she suspected, they were unaware of the problem. A teacher spoke to the girls in the class, telling them how disappointed she was that they were treating each other so terribly. The next day, one of Katie's friends sent her an apology letter and asked if they could play. Gradually, Katie mended her relationships, but Abbe still observes her daughter's behavior to make sure everything is okay.

Imagine how Katie would have continued to suffer if Abbe hadn't followed up on her suspicions that her daughter's panic was emotional. Children's internal crises often manifest themselves physically. Kids start wetting their pants, waking up at night, or getting stomachaches. They may be tired or on edge. It's important for parents not to react negatively to these symptoms, but to investigate possible causes of stress by thinking about changes in the child's life. Even if they can't pinpoint the problem, they can at least take an empathetic stance. Their compassion can help a child feel more sympathetic with his own plight.

Why don't children always come to parents when they are upset or in trouble? Children may not know how to express what they are feeling. They might fear their parents' getting upset or making the situation worse.

Abbe and I agreed that she was able to help Katie because she read between the lines of her daughter's behavior and investigated beyond her daughter's explanations. Her ability to gauge what was happening and inform others without overreacting provided a safety net to allow Katie to express her anguish. At any age, no matter what the problem—tantrums, nightmares, or even alcohol and drugs—sensing a child's reactions and looking past her dismissal of our concerns is one of the best things a parent can do.

One of the most valuable tools for sensing what's actually happening with a child lies in thinking back to the challenges we faced when we were her age.

Did you ever hide problems from your parents? What could they have done to offer the help you needed?

Think Back to Your Childhood

Parenting forces us to get to know ourselves better than we ever might have imagined we could—and in many new ways . . .

FRED ROGERS

When my son, Matt, was fourteen, he fell in love with a darling cheerleader named Lana. Within a few months of constant visits, she felt like part of the family.

Matt had liked girls before, but he had never gone steady. He talked openly about Lana, saying that someday they might be able to marry. That comment took me back to my own adolescent relationship with a tall, good-looking Norwegian neighbor. When we were fourteen we also started going steady and talked about marriage. My father was concerned, but I insisted that the relationship made me happy.

Looking back, however, I realize that I fought my father as part of my teenage rebellion. Underneath, I felt far too young for the pressures of having a boyfriend. I missed hanging out with my girlfriends and talking about boys. I also yearned for the world of play I seemed suddenly to have left behind. I no longer played touch tackle in front of my house. Going steady turned me into a full-fledged teenager who wore her boyfriend's jacket and didn't scrimmage in the street.

Looking at Matt I could see how young a fourteen year old actually is, how much child still exists in the adolescent. Eric Erikson, the renowned psychologist who first outlined stages in the life cycle, described adolescence as a time of forming identity. After the stage of identity comes intimacy. In other words, we have to know who we are before we can have an intimate relationship. By investing in a serious relationship at fourteen, my son was shortchanging himself of the self-defining process. But I only realized this after reflecting on my own past.

One night while Matt and I were doing the dishes, I asked him if he ever found going steady overwhelming. He protested, saying how happy he was with Lana and how much he cared about her. I assured him that I understood. Remembering how I had protested with my father, I talked casually about the pressures I had felt at his age. I wondered aloud if he ever felt that way. Suddenly, Matt began to cry. We talked about experiencing the relationship two different ways—loving Lana and feeling overwhelmed.

Soon after, Matt broke up with Lana and started hanging out with his childhood friends again. He seemed younger and returned to activities like riding his bike. I missed Lana, since I had come to love her, too. But just to prove that destiny has its own way, Matt and Lana happened to meet on a street in San Francisco many years later and started dating again. Today they are happily married and have two children. Since they had had time to fully develop their identities, they found getting to know each other again an exciting, intimate experience.

There was nothing in my son's demeanor that would have cued me to his emotional strain. Remembering my own experience provided the insight. I was lucky that I was able to access those memories at that time, since childhood experiences can be hard to remember. Finding ways of pursuing our childhood feelings—from toddlerhood to our twenties—is one of the best tools for understanding our children.

In her book *Recovery of Your Inner Child*, Lucia Capacchione offers a revolutionary method for tuning in to our childhood emotions that has proved successful with people in all walks of life. She suggests writing a question with one's dominant hand and then answering with the hand one doesn't usually use. When I tried this method to ask the fourteen-year-old child inside of me what she needed then, the answer from my nondominant hand came back, "Understanding." I am grateful that returning to the intense rumblings of my heart as an adolescent allowed me to empathize with my son and to encourage him to develop wisdom about his own needs. I appreciate all the insights about life and the sense of spiritual expansion my relationships with my children have offered me.

Write yourself a question about your feelings at a particular age and answer with your nondominant hand.

Hear Their Spirits

> Grandma said the spirit mind was like any other mus-
> cle. If you used it, it got bigger and stronger. She said
> the only way it could get that way was using it to
> understand . . . and the more you tried to understand,
> the bigger it got.
>
>

FORREST CARTER

When my daughter Gabrielle was five, I was driving children home
from school in our car pool one day. A boy in Gabrielle's kindergarten
class named Willy seemed sad about something that had happened at
school. Finally, he exclaimed, "I hate myself." There was a moment of
silence, then Gabrielle turned to him in distress and said, "Don't ever
say you hate yourself, Willy. It upsets God." She paused as if she were
trying to explain something very difficult. "He wants us to love ourselves because He's inside us. If you say you hate yourself, you are hat-
ing God. So try and love yourself." Willy was stunned and didn't speak
the rest of the way to his house. So was I.

Later, I realized I had forgotten to ask Willy what he was sad about. I
was too shocked by my daughter's convictions about what God wants.
Where had they come from? Not from me. We had talked about God, but
I still didn't know how to love myself, nor had I linked God to feelings
about ourselves. Why was my five-year-old daughter speaking about our
sacred duty not to offend God by putting ourselves down? Gabrielle had
obviously been trying to understand some spiritual truths, and her conclusions emerged from nothing she had learned at home or at school.

Spiritual truths don't have to be about God. I still remember the day I asked my three-year-old son why he was crying, probably with a tone that implied it wasn't necessary. My son turned to me and spoke with conviction. "You know it's fine to cry, Mom," he said. "There's nothing wrong with it. Crying can be good." Again, recognizing his words as truth I changed my whole perspective and apologized for my impatience.

I have talked to countless parents about the surprisingly wise things their children say and how they react to them. "You know it's the wise old man inside of Sam," one mother told me. "He has that deep knowing part that pops out sometimes in what he says." More and more parents I talk to take that perspective. They believe that even though their children exhibit all the traits of being three, six, or eight years old, they also have an internal voice that seems ageless. It's up to us to encourage their attempts to struggle with the secrets of life. One father said, "My father still remembers the wise things I said when I was young. That part of us gets covered up if no one pays attention to it."

How do we encourage the spiritual knowing of children? Our media address our children as budding consumers. Books on child rearing want to equip us to raise our children's IQ, help them to make more friends, and turn them into athletic or musical virtuosos. Our society tends to ignore the spirits of our children, unless we are trying to instruct them on what they should believe. We don't have to believe in God to value our child's developing a full perspective on life's meaning. Parents today are more likely to listen to their children's thoughts and have two-sided conversations about the deeper sides of life.

Recently, four-year-old Araceli drew a picture of a beautiful figure with rainbow colors and said, "This is my guardian angel. She's with me all the time." When I told her mother, Aida, she said Araceli talks to her about the angel at nighttime. Aida even suggested that Araceli try to find out the angel's name when she goes to sleep. I love this mother's respect for her daughter's spiritual interests and the wonder that they share in their discussions of all the seen and unseen mysteries of life. Parents like Aida believe that listening to their children's spiritual perceptions at each stage helps their "spirit mind," mentioned in the opening quote, to grow. When we pay attention to that growth and make talking about it part of family life, we strengthen our abilities to know each other.

What places, activities, and parts of life seemed magical to you as a child? What beliefs about life's mysteries did you ruminate on?

CHAPTER 8

Make Family Matter

Create Cooperation

Definition: To cooperate—to work with another or to associate with another for mutual benefit.

My mother's passion is knitting. Sometimes she has been paid for her designs, but more often she makes them to satisfy her own creativity then gives them away. As a child, I would help my mother in the evenings, winding balls of yarn. It took lots of concentration, and seeing the exquisitely colored balls pile up around us gave me a feeling of beauty and accomplishment. I also liked working with my father on projects like building a small stone wall in our garden. There was something about doing it with him that I loved.

As the definition that begins this chapter reveals, cooperation occurs when two people work interdependently toward a common goal, a different kind of labor from tackling a project on our own. As a child, I resisted having to wash the dishes or being sent to clean up my room. I honed my arguments about not having time for chores so well that my father humorously suggested I become a lawyer. Yet I enjoyed working with either of my parents on projects.

I never thought much about my fondness for these cooperative activities until years later, when I participated for several years in a women's group. During a particular phase, we drew pictures of childhood activities and shared them. When asked to depict a favorite activity, I was amazed that almost every one of us drew ourselves working on a project with a parent, like baking cookies or gardening.

My husband tells me that he loved waxing a car with one of his favorite father figures. "It seemed like a grown-up thing to do." I think part of the pleasure of shared work is that the adult sees the child as having the competence for collaboration and wishes to include him in the activity.

Learning to work together is an acquired skill that we need throughout our lives. In the past, children learned cooperation through myriad activities in which people—adults and children— worked together: picking berries, sewing quilts, putting on a new roof, painting the house, making ornaments, or cooking a pie. Today we have to remember to include children in our tasks because of the pressure to do things quickly. As one mother told me, "I purposely include my son, but I have to plan that when we do a project together it will take three times as long as doing it on my own."

Our lives are so overscheduled that research shows cooperative abilities in children are actually in danger of extinction. For several years, I worked as a consultant to the Child Development Project, then located in San Ramon, California, which is dedicated to finding ways social skills such as cooperating can be instilled in children today. The project's research has shown that one of the best things parents can do is take the time to peel carrots, fold clothes, or clean the kitchen with their child. The more children engage in cooperative activities, the more motivated they become to help and work with others harmoniously.

I learned that in my own life. When my children were about twelve, ten, and four, we rushed through after-dinner tasks with lots of squabbling about who should do what. Monitoring whether they finished their chores was additional work for me, so I tried something new. A dear friend suggested we institute a "family work hour." For one hour after dinner, we worked, usually in pairs or groups of three, on things that needed to be done. At first the children resisted, but after a while they started coming up with ideas for projects we could do. We had some of our best conversations while we worked. The kids also became more and more helpful. Looking back, our joint projects are some of my favorite memories of that time period. I still enjoy working side by side with my children on projects, now that they are adults. The pleasure has lasted.

Isn't it nice to think that when we cook with a child or shine silver, we are not only developing closeness, we are setting a template for the way cooperation and satisfying work feel? When we step out of pressured time, working or playing, we experience what psychologists call "flow," the ability to lose ourselves in our actions. Our children can take that harmony, skill, and ability to flow into activity with them into their own families.

Draw a picture of work that you enjoyed doing with an adult, when you were a child, or that you like doing with your child now.

A Picnic Is Worth the Time It Takes

Spend the afternoon; you can't take it with you.

ANNIE DILLARD

One of my hairdressers, Jeffrey, immigrated to California from London fifteen years ago, but he is still unable to understand our approach to relaxation. "In England, when I made a plan to do something for the afternoon, like a picnic, I left the time open-ended. We would have a picnic at noon and let the pleasure of the experience extend as far into the day as it naturally would. In the States, people chop their relaxation into chunks of time. My friend plans to play tennis with one person in the morning, meet another for lunch at noon, do yardwork in the afternoon, and then have someone else over to dinner. I just can't enjoy life that way."

Jeffrey's description of unscheduled pleasure reminds me of the way I approached having fun as a child. Do you remember playing outside after dinner in summer and wishing that the half-glow evening light would last forever? When my friends and I planned to go swimming, we didn't calculate how long it would take us to pack our suits, get them on, swim, dry off, and get back home to do something else. All we imagined and experienced were the pleasure of the water and each other's company. When adults could join us in that fun mode, it was even better. Some of my happiest memories are of afternoons swimming with my father—a time when he let go of responsibilities—and the feeling of timelessness, floating on the Russian River together.

At what point do we start planning pleasure into tight little packages? Our culture teaches us to calculate the time and trouble that a proposed pleasurable experience might be worth—an hour for lunch with a friend, an hour at the park with our child after work, because we promised. For a parent who works full time outside the home, being able to go to the park after work for an hour is highly commendable. But keeping our eyes on our watch keeps us from losing ourselves in the experience. Chronicling the time means part of us is always absent from the event. The relaxation we all long for comes only with complete absorption in the delight of the activity, only when we step out of our consciousness of time.

On a hot weekend day last August, my son and I hatched a plan to take his children swimming. It took lots of preparation to pack all the right accessories for a two year old and an eight month old to get wet, dry off, drink, and eat as needed. When we finally got to the pool, our schedule allowed us only a very short time to swim. However, as we held them, giggling, in the water, something magical happened. We didn't want to leave. The original plan dictated getting the children home for their naps "on time." We postponed the naps, which finally took place at my house, and we then had an unplanned dinner together. As we extended enjoyment into the evening, I began to feel like the child who didn't want it to get dark. I could see from their expressions that my grandchildren and son felt the same way.

In 2002, the Boys and Girls Clubs of America in Atlanta published a study based on interviews with parents and children about what constitutes quality time. Not surprisingly, the two groups differed in their perspectives. Sharing an activity wasn't enough for the children; they wanted adults to have fun doing it! Having the attitude that enjoyment is worth the time it takes is one of the best things parents can do. When parents really play, they join children and participate with them in the joy of life—what the French call *joie de vivre*. Even if we only have twenty minutes, we can let go of everything other than the moment. But occasionally we need to really "spend" the afternoon and relinquish it to its most pleasurable conclusion if we want our children to continue to enjoy our company.

With that goal in mind, we can turn our home into an environment where our children and their friends love to come.

> **List some enjoyable childhood experiences when you never wanted the day to end. Hang your list on the refrigerator to remind yourself that you and your family need to lose yourselves in fun moments whenever possible.**

Host Open House

Look well to the hearthstone; there hope
for America lies.

CALVIN COOLIDGE

The night Rob and Loel hosted the high-school football team at their home for a "night-before-the-game-pasta feed," the team members arrived covered with mud. They had practiced during the first rain of the season. Loel handed out every towel in the house to get the guys dry. The football players eventually gathered on the roofed deck outside to consume about three hotdogs and half a pound of pasta each. After devouring all they could, the boys retired to an outside room to have their ritual talk about tomorrow's game. Meanwhile, Loel heard scratching at the front door and opened it to see her dog staring at her whimpering in pain. At first Loel thought his head had shrunk. Then she realized that his stomach was about four times its usual size. "He looked as if someone had blown his stomach up with a bicycle pump. Then I realized he had gotten in the garbage can and eaten all the scraps of hot dog and pasta. It was so sad." Loel put the dog in the car and drove him to get his stomach pumped.

Despite the fact that she had a lot of cleanup waiting at home, there were no towels left in the linen closet, and the storm had knocked out the stoplights on the way to the veterinarian, she felt the evening was worth it. As one of the football players said as he departed, "I want my house to be just like this when I'm grown up."

Loel was touched, since she assumed he meant a house that was a relaxed place for kids to hang out. She and Rob have worked hard to make their house a place where their sons and their friends gather.

What makes a home a place where kids want to come? Letting the kids feel comfortable and nourished, say Rob and Loel. Loel remembers coming home one day to find Rob playing hockey with the boys on their hardwood floor. "I realized then that we might have a nice house but that it was never going to be perfect," she says. "Our solution was to make places for the boys to go with their friends. First we converted the garage to a playroom, and then we built a separate room outside. It's shaped like a yurt, so the kids love it." She also admits their food bill is usually enormous, since the kids' friends eat over so often.

If the suburbs offer few places for kids to go, the city overflows with activity, but much of it unwholesome. Like Loel and Rob, Dameon's father, Steve, placed a high priority on kids coming over to the house. Dameon attended, an urban high school, and his friends were diverse racially and economically. When kids gathered at his house, Steve often found himself playing the role of mediator about disputes that had arisen during the day. He says he encouraged open communication and provided a supportive, nonjudgmental space for such openness. Over time, Steve's house became a port in the storm for Dameon's friends. He says he became close to the kids as "father, uncle, big brother, and teacher figure."

If we want to have an influence on kids, we have to be around them and hear what's happening in their lives. Hosting open house means more work, but many parents—myself included—feel that providing a safe, supervised place for young people is one of the best things they can do. As we listen to young people's interests, we also have the chance to share our own values and the activities we love, a process that keeps our connections current and strong.

Was there an adult other than your parent that you liked being around, when you were young? How did spending time with that person help you? As a teenager, how did you feel about bringing friends home?

Share Your Passions

Imagine what a harmonious world it could be if every single person, both young and old, shared a little of what he is good at doing.

QUINCY JONES

Diane Frolov and Andy Schneider, Emmy-award-winning writers and producers of successful TV shows such as *Northern Exposure, Alien Nation,* and *Dangerous Minds,* have shared their passions with their son, Joseph, since he was a little boy.

When Joseph was young they brought him to their group dance class. Joseph played airplanes and watched couples practicing the foxtrot and waltz. At fourteen, Joseph started taking lessons in the same class as his parents, and the teacher found him quite talented. As a teenager, Joseph discovered he had caught his parents' passion for ballroom dancing and went on to enter competitions.

They also shared their love of script writing and the filmmaking process. They spent months with Joseph on the set of *Northern Exposure* in the wilds of Washington State. When Joseph was older, the three of them formed a "movie club." Diane and Andy introduced Joseph to their favorite films from the seventies, on video, discussing the aspects they loved of each movie. Now Joseph is a theater major at UCLA and has also studied creative writing. Diane and Andy's commitment to sharing their love of the arts with him has provided him with vibrant examples of how people can use their talents and passions with inspiration and joy. He has also been able to observe their perseverance when scripts or shows didn't work out, revealing how resilient people in the industry have to be.

When parents invite their children into their passions, kids see how interesting and demanding pouring oneself into an activity can be. On the other hand, sharing can go both ways.

My friend Maggie loves classical music and has listened to it for years with her son Bobby. When he wanted to turn the radio to heavy metal and later rap as they drove to junior high each morning, she surprised herself by agreeing to listen.

Maggie says they were both intrigued by the roots of rap music. She discovered that some of the artists showed real genius. Sometimes, she liked lyrics that were particularly "from the heart," but, just as often, she felt revulsion. She could have tuned out in these cases, or followed the example of many parents who shouted, "Turn off that crap!" Instead, she seized the opportunity to engage with Bobby on his own terms.

"Does what they are saying bother you?" she would ask, and often it did upset him. Those free-ranging discussions were a medium for talking to Bobby about all kinds of issues that might not have come up if Maggie had rejected his music. Now he is in college, and their listening sessions have continued. Meanwhile, Bobby's tastes have expanded to include many types of music, and he even takes voice lessons.

In the quote that begins this chapter, Quincy Jones makes the outrageous suggestion that if young and old talked about what they are good at doing, the world would be more harmonious. I think he is on to something. Imagine what life could be like if parents and children agreed to share their passions, like countries participating in a cultural exchange. How lively and informative our communication would be! As adults, we know better than to adopt our children's interests as our own, but sharing helps us to know each other better.

List ten things you love to do, then ten things your child loves to do. Do you take time as a family to honor both?

PART III

The BeST THiNGs PaRENTS DO for TheMSeLVEs

Now we will journey on to discuss the crucial role of caring for ourselves. The world too often tears people down, and the demands of our lives wear us out. "How to" books describe "right" ways to parent, and the people in their hypothetical examples always know what to do.

One of the best things we can do as parents is to stop comparing ourselves to ideals and look at ourselves as learners who, above all, have to believe we can meet life's challenges. Being a learner allows us to feel humble rather than lacking, open to change rather than anxious and guilt-ridden.

Caring for a child is the most important job in the world. To meet the daily demands of this job, we must not ignore ourselves. We are the only ones who can identify our strengths and take care of our bodies. Few people will insist that we take the time we need to rest and recharge ourselves. No one is going to manage our stress or keep our mood light. We need to know when we need a few minutes—or a whole weekend—away. It's up to us to sense when our relationship with our child seems out of balance and we need to get some advice.

When we concentrate on being kind to ourselves and recharging our spiritual and physical energy, we cope with challenges more effectively and enjoy the moment more. We also provide role models of self-confidence and self-care for our children.

Caring for ourselves is one of the best things we can do because our child's happiness and productivity revolve around our well-being. We can't afford to let ourselves or our children down.

CHAPTER 9

Take Good Care of Yourself

Find Islands of Peace

When you're experiencing peace, it's coming from within you, you're doing peace.

CHERI HUBER AND JUNE SHIVER

Bonnie could hardly speak, she was so upset. Tears shone in her eyes, and she held her hand over her mouth as if to keep from screaming. I could tell it had been one of those mornings. I waited until she calmed herself. "Is there anything I can do?" I asked.

She drew a deep breath. "The last few mornings it's been horrible getting the boys to school. They aren't listening, and I've ended up yelling and then feeling helpless and guilty. We all hate each other by the time we leave the house. I really feel like I'm falling down on the job as a mom."

If I hadn't observed, many times, the way stress can color a parent's thinking, I would have been shocked by Bonnie's self-assessment. She does more after-school activities with her boys than any parent I know and is always concerned about being sensitive to their needs.

That's why it was apparent to me that Bonnie wasn't "falling down" or failing as a mother—she was falling down in taking care of herself. In the book *Time-Out . . . for Parents: A Compassionate Approach to Parenting*, Cheri Huber and Melinda Guyol say that when we "lose it" and start shouting at our kids, something within us is signaling loud and clear that it's been neglected. When we are tired from giving to others and not looking at our own needs, it's almost impossible to think in a balanced way. We lack the reserves for self-control.

Bonnie and I talked about self-nurturance, and not long after that she took advantage of a women's weekend retreat and came back refreshed. She also started volunteering weekly at her children's school office—an activity she really enjoys. She's back to looking like that courageous mom I know.

Time away is great for recharging our spirits, but it's still not the whole picture. Learning to create peace in the midst of activity is one of the best things a parent can do. We need to recoup internally even when children are begging for another cookie or fighting over a train. When we suppress angry feelings rather than acknowledging or dealing with them, we're more likely to explode. If we can learn to "do peace" even once, while surrounded by chaos, it develops our ability to do it again and again.

The authors of *Time-Out* recommend stopping and taking deep breaths: "As you breathe, allow your attention to move into your body with your breath: Where is the tension? . . .'What am I feeling?' . . . Simply be present in this moment, just noticing." Going inside allows us to be present to ourselves so that we can recover from outer bombardment.

How do we take an internal minivacation while our children are screaming? We can sit down and close our eyes and say, "I need a minute to rest." I also love Rudolf Dreikurs' advice to parents in *Children: The Challenge*: Go into the bathroom and play the radio with the door locked. Closing ourselves off for even few minutes lets children know we need a "time-out."

Another method I've discovered for reaching inside for calm in the midst of crisis is using positive imagery. When I'm working with a screaming child, I often picture myself on a tropical island with a warm, white sand beach, so that my peaceful feelings can rise and soothe us both.

When you feel as if you are falling down as a parent, take that as a sign that you need to care for yourself the same way you would care for a tired child. Stopping helps us and our children, because if we keep going we can exhaust our "giving supply." Tell yourself that inner peace is just a deep breath away and that you always have a beautiful island beach within you. After you take that fantasy vacation, remind yourself of all the positive things you do and applaud yourself for them.

Draw a picture of what "doing peace" means to you and hang it in a place where you can easily refer to it.

Applaud Your Own Efforts

It is up to us to give ourselves recognition. . . . When you do something you are proud of, dwell on it a little, praise yourself for it, relish the experience, take it in. . . . When things go wrong, they call attention to themselves. When things go well, we must actively hold them in our attention.

MILDRED NEWMAN AND BERNARD BERKOWITZ

It took months for Margo to help her four-year-old son Sean to have more self-control about hitting his friends, and his growth didn't occur because he moved on to a new stage. Margo coached Sean to talk when he was angry rather than hitting. (Say, "I'm angry that you grabbed my truck.") I watched Sean hold his hands at his side like a soldier at attention while he poured out his frustration. Talking with Margo, I mentioned how important I thought it was for her to pat herself on the back for her accomplishment with Sean. She shrugged her shoulders as if I were joking. Why is it that applauding ourselves as parents feels silly?

At work we often get positive feedback on a project well done. We also can get awards in a weight-loss program for pounds lost. We probably wouldn't shrug off a compliment about the results of our efforts in any other arena. But parenting is an activity that rarely involves a feeling of closure or accomplishment, except vicariously when our children win at a sports event or receive an award. How can we measure our success unless we become aware of our goals and acknowledge the efforts we make toward realizing them?

Marking the times when we have helped our child with a problem or supported her in an important way gives us a sense of our own effectiveness. When new challenges arise, we can remind ourselves that we have learned to overcome hurdles in the past, and we can do it again. Dwelling on our accomplishment of the hour, day, or month is like rooting for our favorite team. As parents we need all the encouragement we can get. We function better when we feel strong. "Go! Go! You're doing great!"

Margo's work to help her son manage his aggression wasn't a little thing. Sean angers easily and reacts possessively with toys. Learning to contain his anger is a great big step in his development and will affect his future relationships and the lives of others who are close to him. Perhaps one of the reasons that we pay little attention to the ways we help our children is that we don't know that their development could have gone in another direction if we hadn't intervened. Is Margo aware that without her consistent efforts Sean could still be pushing and shoving other children in first and second grade? Does she know that his lack of self-control would have affected his ability to make friends? We need to recognize the importance of the help we give our children toward positive development, noticing little successes as well as big ones.

In addition to applauding our own efforts, it's helpful to observe the accomplishments of other parents. Even if the world doesn't notice, we can commend each other's efforts and provide needed encouragement. Our praise can help others to appreciate themselves. The more we support one another in doing a good job, the better job we'll all do.

The quotation that starts this chapter, urging us to dwell on what we are proud of, is from the bestselling book *How to Be Your Own Best Friend*. In this slim volume, Newman and Berkowitz point out how much we all resist feeling good about what we do, and how much unhappiness we create by our resistance to treating ourselves kindly. We owe it to our kids, ourselves, and other parents to cheer for the work we all do and to feel that cheering matters—that it's one of the best things we can do. We owe it to ourselves to believe in our strengths and to remember that it often takes a crisis to identify what they are.

Make a list of your accomplishments as a parent. Create stickies to put on mirrors and on the refrigerator, noting changes and congratulating yourself on your efforts.

Notice Your Wonderful Strengths

No one can appreciate me to the degree I deserve. . . .
For as much as someone may value what I offer, no one
knows what it took for me to become the person I am, to
be able to offer what I have."

RONALD MAH, M.A.

Today Rosemary is a shining example and resource for other parents, but when I first met her she was completely overwhelmed. She had just given birth to her third son, and her two-and-a-half-year-old son, Patrick, had been diagnosed with Asperger's syndrome. Rosemary was shocked because her pediatrician had always regarded Patrick's development as normal. Asperger's, a milder form of autism, is often identified late in children, even up to age nine, because their problems with social interaction don't stand out when they are very young. Patrick had good language development, but Rosemary didn't realize that his speech wasn't conversational.

"I was so confused," she remembers. "I had never heard of Asperger's, and I had no idea what to do. I certainly wasn't going to talk to other people about this new challenge with my son. I didn't even tell my parents about the diagnosis for two months."

Rosemary left her high-paying job as a defense attorney and started to learn about Asperger's. She admits that in the beginning she was still in denial. She would read about miracle cures and try them out, including putting Patrick on a casein/gluten-free diet and having him listen to certain kinds of music. None of these interventions produced any results. In the process, however, Rosemary began to apply the strengths that she'd had all her life to this new challenge with Patrick.

"As a trial lawyer, I have very strong organizational abilities and the capacity to analyze," she told me. "I am accustomed to advocating for my client in a very objective way while remaining friendly with the opposing attorney. I have had to learn not to take things personally and to be very creative and tenacious. All of those strengths have been perfect for what I have needed to do for Patrick."

Reading everything she could find on Asperger's and contacting support groups turned Rosemary into an expert on providing the best educational program for her son. She hired tutors and advocated to get help for him from the school district. Today he is attending kindergarten in public school and progressing in his social and academic skills.

The school district now refers parents with similar problems to Rosemary. She talks them through the process of getting their children the services they need. That's where all her analytic abilities come into play. In the future, she wants to provide free legal assistance for parents of special-needs children who want to get help for their children.

It would have been easy for Rosemary to fall into a self-deprecating cycle after Patrick's diagnosis. In her affluent community, where high achievement is revered, some people treated her differently once they knew she had a special-needs child. What if she had concentrated on the hardships of having an Asperger's child or told herself how helpless she was to affect his life? There is no doubt that homing in on her strengths to deal with the challenge was the path of growth for Rosemary.

It doesn't have to take a crisis for us to think about our past accomplishments and identify the marvelous strengths that can help us as parents. But approaching challenges with an "I can do!" attitude opens our perspectives. Like Rosemary, we do our best when we concentrate on our capabilities. From a place of strength, we can even occasionally laugh at the challenging situations life provides for us.

What are your strengths and how did you acquire them? In challenging situations, what abilities do you use?

Laugh Your Cares Away

If I were given the opportunity to give a gift to the next generation, it would be the ability for each individual to learn to laugh at himself.

CHARLES SCHULZ

Amanda heard singing coming from her bedroom, and the lyrics made her a little anxious: "The moment I wake up, I put on my makeup." Curious, she peered through the door and gasped. Her two-year-old daughter was standing with the stub of a lipstick in her hand. Her face was smeared with lipstick, and there was red all over the mirrored doors of the closets, the wall, and who knows where else. Amanda closed the door, walked down the hall, and sat on the stairs with her head in her hands. She had to take a few minutes or her anger would explode. But when she thought of her daughter singing that song, she laughed. "Looking at the funny side of situations saves my mood and preserves my health. The things you have to put up with as a parent are so bizarre that you could be exploding all the time, and that's not helpful to me or them."

I still tell about the day I had to take my six-year-old son's mouse to the veterinarian, even though I had the stomach flu. Matt cried in the morning because the mouse seemed sick, and I promised I would get the mouse treated. In the vet's office I had to hold the mouse while the doctor gave him a shot. However, the tiny creature jumped from my hand, and I chased him around the office while the doctor stood poised with the injection needle in midair. It was hard not to vomit.

When my son came home from school, I called out the good news from my sickbed. "Mousie will get better," I yelled. My son yelled, "Great!" and ran outside to play. I could have gotten angry that he didn't stop to look in on me or on Mousie, but getting angry would have escalated my nausea so I chose to think of the craziness and laugh.

Laughing at ourselves and the ridiculous situations we find ourselves in is one of the best ways of coping with the insanity of parenthood. Pulling apart two children trying to choke each other can propel us into a screaming rage or uproarious laughter at the physical risks of being a referee. If we take our own plight lightly, we will be better equipped to change our child's mood and perpetuate our good feelings. We might start counting like a referee to break up a fight between young children and get our numbers mixed up: "One, two, forty-six, and fifty-five." Young children love to make fun of our mistakes.

In fact, if we can remember to use humor, we are more likely to preserve our well-being and health. Just smiling increases blood flow to the brain and stimulates positive neurotransmitters. In controlled studies, humor raised pain thresholds, reduced stress, and boosted immune function. Getting angry, on the other hand, pumps adrenaline into the bloodstream, making us want to fight or flee. It can propel us into fighting with our children or withdrawing from them.

Laughing at ourselves or at situations also helps us maintain a healthy connection with our child. Parents who work at getting a child to laugh will get into far fewer power struggles. When Laurie's young son would scream for an ice cream cone on the way home, she would say, "I want one too. I want the biggest ice cream cone in the whole world. I want an ice cream cone as big as a mountain." Her son would stop screaming and picture the gigantic cone. The technique of exaggerating how we would like to fulfill the child's wish, even though we can't at that moment, allows us to align with him emotionally.

Whenever we laugh with a child (or another adult), our energy blends with theirs, and our thoughts are freed like birds to fly in more positive directions.

Parenthood requires monumental, silent sacrifices and tremendous acts of love and self-control. Why not laugh along the way?

Are there any funny stories that are part of the lore of the family you grew up in? What kinds of things did you laugh about? How do you remind yourself to see the humorous side of situations now?

PART IV

THe BeST THiNGs PaReNTS DO for EaCh OthER

It seems to me that one of the pivotal things we can learn to do is approach each other with compassion and work together for the benefit of children—not just our kids, but everyone's. Our common basis for supporting each other isn't that we have the same lifestyles or religious beliefs, but that we have been entrusted with the care of the next generation. We have a chance to make a difference in their lives, and that's the biggest gift we can bequeath to the future.

Our materialistic society encourages subtle competition between parents. It's easy to be envious of a parent who can buy his child more things. It's hard not to feel competitive with someone whose child has better grades or achieves higher SAT scores, because that's what our society values. But in our complex age neither possessions, nor good grades, nor high test scores are indicators of the person a child will become. We live in a time of such varied influences and values that parents can't afford comparison and competition. The only way we can protect children's prized potentials is to work together cooperatively, rising above the illusory divisions of "my child" and "your child."

My heart is warmed every day by the support and understanding I see shared by people who care about children. Whether others believe as we do or handle issues the same way, we all need help to do our best in our roles caring for children. Looking for new ways to help each other is one of the best things we can do to make life better for families now and in generations to come.

CHAPTER 10

Build Bridges to the Future

Put Yourself in Their Shoes

It is one of the most beautiful compensations of life,
that no man can sincerely try to help another without
helping himself.

RALPH WALDO EMERSON

Enjoying an evening by herself is a rare treat for Ann. Her ex-husband
Allen travels for work and doesn't often have the opportunity to take
their son Abe overnight. One such night the phone rang, just as she
was getting in the bathtub. Ann was dismayed to see Allen's number
on the caller ID. She wondered if Abe were sick. "I was even more
upset when I heard what Allen had to say. He started calling Abe a brat,
because he couldn't get him into bed. Abe isn't used to staying at his
Dad's, so he was scared. Allen didn't know what to do, so he wanted to
bring Abe back."

Ann could hardly contain her rage. She had been so flexible about
adjusting the visitation schedule to fit Allen's needs, and now he
wanted to rob her of her only evening alone at home. Couldn't he
show a little understanding? She was a breath away from berating him
as a terrible father when she thought about the question she had just
asked herself about Allen. Could she just show him "a little understanding"? As Ben Franklin once said, you get more flies with honey
than vinegar.

As a salesperson, Ann is a highly skilled communicator. She has
always found offering sympathy helpful, even to her ex-husband. This
time her efforts had an immediate effect. "I know getting Abe in bed

can be daunting. It's a real hassle for me sometimes, too." Allen stopped his tirade and started asking questions about what to do. Ann and Allen ended up talking for about a half hour, sharing ideas and commiserating with each other about the challenges of parenting. "I couldn't believe things turned around so quickly and easily. The conversation helped both of us. I really want Abe, and Allen to have a good relationship, and unloading my anger would have been disastrous." Their mutual understanding will help Abe, too. "Since I want Allen to be a good father, I've tried to think about what qualities he has that will be helpful to Abe. When I can remember to reach out to him with sympathy, I've seen that it brings those qualities out."

This isn't the first time I've been impressed with Ann's ability to approach her ex-husband with a higher purpose in mind. In this instance, not expressing her criticism of Allen prevented him from feeling like an incompetent father and giving up. Admitting her own problems with their son at bedtime allowed them to talk as equals—helping to create a foundation for co-parenting in the future. Her efforts remind me of a quote from the Buddhist scriptures:

> One in all,
> All in One.
> If only that is realized.
> No more worry about not being perfect.

Creating a bridge that modifies our thinking about good and bad, higher or lower, right and wrong is one of the most productive things we can do with others. Offering understanding to her ex-husband in spite of all his mistakes, past and present, makes their relationship less competitive and more cooperative. Ann doesn't have to be the perfect parent who knows everything and tries to get her child's father to shape up. They are both just people trying to learn about raising a child.

One of the best things we can do as parents is admit our mistakes and accept others' weaknesses out of a higher regard for what happens with our child. Our ability to understand the teacher's view on students' responsibilities or the babysitter's need to be heard is often the key to working together successfully. Our opinion that the teacher requires too much homework, or the babysitter allows behavior we want to extinguish, doesn't need to make our conversations adversarial. We can listen to others' concerns with the understanding that each of us sees a child from a different perspective, then build a bridge that isn't based on ideas of right and wrong, to reach out to each other as compassionate human beings.

Think of someone whose view of child rearing is different from yours, and list that person's good qualities.

Reach Out for Guidance

No Man is an Island, entire of itself.

JOHN DONNE

When Michael heard that he was going to be a father, he was thrilled. Learning that his wife, Caryl, was expecting twins, however, overwhelmed him. His first conscious thought was, "I'm going to need help." Michael wasn't sure what kind of help he had in mind, but after a few months an idea emerged. He wanted to have a party—a kind of transition-to-fatherhood party for himself—that would help him feel confident about being a dad.

At the party, there were grandfathers, stepfathers, fathers of twins, and fathers of children of all ages. The men were anxious to talk and offer their advice. "Two points of view emerged, and they have both proven helpful to me," he told me. "One was to be involved with my kids in every way possible—teach them, play with them, guide them, investigate the world with them—and that's mainly the kind of father I have been. The other point of view was to follow your passion as far as the work you choose, and everything will be fine with your children because you will be doing what you love and feel authentic."

Michael's twins are now seven, and he is constantly involved in activities with them. They garden, build things, observe animals and birds, cook, and have consistent play times. Michael admits that the second point of view expressed by the men has also helped him. His job has been more demanding than he ever anticipated, and when he has to be away from his children he remembers men he respects saying, "You also have to do what you love, and everything will be okay."

When Michael thinks back to the event he created, he feels grateful in ways that are hard to put into words. "I wanted to have a party that would honor fatherhood and say that it's important in itself—an event that would make fathers feel good about their roles. I don't see how it's possible to realize your ideals as a father without knowing how others do it. I had the meeting with the hope it would start a tradition of fathers connecting to one another. We haven't done it formally since then, but I do talk to the other dads pretty frequently and share stories."

Whenever parents reach out to each other, they get more than the specific advice they asked for. They become aware, if they let themselves, that parenting isn't something that they are doing alone. The men who came to Michael's house were eager to share because there are few venues for men to express the ways they have stretched themselves to be dads. We hear every day about how much mothers have to balance demands, but we don't hear very much about men and the dramatic changes in their roles.

Reaching out to someone for guidance is a way of acknowledging that we are learners. Whether we talk to our mom, our sister, our friend, or a professional, we are saying, "We think better collectively, and I'm not afraid to admit I need help. If we talk, maybe we can plan how to handle things better."

In these men's minds, being a father probably provided some of the most important learning experiences in their lives. By connecting with each other, they were saying, "We share these ideals, and we will support each other in reaching for them." Their affirmation of one another as people eager to learn reminds me of a line from a Robert Frost poem, "Men work together whether they work together or apart."

Who are the people you reach out to for guidance? List them in order of the quality of support each offers you.

Make a Plan Together

**No two people see things in exactly the same way.
Mindfulness gives respect to the sovereignty of each
person's unique mind.**

DANIEL SIEGEL, M.D. AND MARY HARTZELL, M.ED.

When Laura and John moved into a new neighborhood, they were delighted to learn there was another boy their son Daniel's age across the street. Edward and Daniel started spending time at each other's homes from the day they moved in. But it was not long before Laura discovered that the two families had dramatically different views about TV. "We were shocked that Edward's family had the TV on all the time. We don't allow Daniel to watch TV, only videos. When Daniel went over to play, he'd often end up watching for hours."

Laura could have refused to let Daniel go to his new friend's house, but wisely she didn't handle the issue that way. Her idea was to contact Edward's mother, Sue, and make a plan. When they got together, she told Sue that Daniel had been adversely affected by TV when he was about four. He became aggressive with his friends after watching, and so they made the difficult decision of removing TV from their house. By framing the situation as her own problem with Daniel, Laura felt that Sue was less likely to feel threatened or judged by their concerns.

Sue seemed open to problem solving and explained her own point of view. She and her husband had felt that TV calmed Edward and that he needed a downtime just to rest. She wanted Daniel to be able to visit without watching TV and suggested they could send Daniel home at times when Edward needed to relax. Most times, they would turn off the TV when Daniel arrived.

Compromising to make a plan isn't always easy, but the plan that Laura and Sue made lasted for years. As adolescents the boys have remained good friends. These parents proved that when people refuse to polarize themselves, everyone benefits.

I am convinced that one important key to this kind of communication is expecting and respecting differences. Parents can get upset when their neighbors, spouses, or babysitters see things differently than they do. I almost never see a situation related to children, however, when people's perceptions don't vary. Today we have the chance to enhance our understanding through talking and working together in compassionate ways. Making a plan is one of the best things people can do to work together effectively.

To plan, we need to look at the dynamics of a situation objectively, deciding what positive solutions we can agree on. Planning allows us to anticipate situations and respond in balanced ways. While we were visiting some friends, our hosts told my husband and me how they had stuck to their plan of not extending their teenager's curfew the night before, even though she argued with them for three hours. Planning allowed them to stand strong.

Once we've arrived at an understanding of what we want, our plan gives us mental clarity and strength to carry out what we believe. Planning with others also helps break down our traditional ideas of what being related means. We develop concern for other children and broaden our conception of family.

What points can you and your partner, or someone who shares the care of your child, agree on?
Write a list of the differing values you and another parent or caregiver bring to the table, and describe how you have learned to work together.

Expand Your Idea of Family

Each of us must come to care about everyone else's
children. We must recognize that the welfare of our
children is intimately linked to the welfare of all other
people's children. . . . The good life for our own children
can be secured only if a good life is also secured for all
other people's children.

LILIAN KATZ

Bonnie was aware that Tom's father had an alcohol problem even
before Tom called to say he had run away because his father had
threatened him physically. Tom and Bonnie's son Derek had been
friends since grade school, and Bonnie could tell Tom had been feeling lost for a long time. They picked Tom up in a park; he had no
clothes nor any possessions with him. Luckily, in Bonnie's county the
law allows people to take in runaway teenagers with impunity.
Bonnie offered to let Tom stay with her family, which included two
sons and two daughters.

Tom's parents were divorced, and Bonnie knew that Tom wasn't
doing well, going back and forth between his mom's house and his
dad's. "Some people get angry and say, 'This isn't fair,' and fight.
Others kind of curl up inside. That was Tom. I knew he was very intelligent and talented, but he was cutting school and giving up. He didn't
want to play the system. I wanted Tom to have the chance he needed,"
Bonnie said. Tom's mother went to court and got sole custody of her
son. She was thankful to have Tom live with Bonnie's family.

Overnight, Bonnie expanded her family and started working on giving Tom the structure she felt he needed. She told him he had to go to school full time or work full time, or do each half time. He also had to help with chores around the house like everyone else, and he couldn't use alcohol or drugs. Tom agreed, and although he was confused, he seemed to sense that being there was a good thing. Bonnie and her husband were happy to offer Tom free room and board if he abided by their conditions. "We were both working, so it wasn't a hardship for us," she said. "My attitude was that if I had the resources to help him, I should do it, because his parents couldn't afford to contribute much at that time."

Bonnie made sure that Tom did his homework every night. She didn't know if he would ever graduate from his independent high school, but she was convinced he needed that encouragement. One day he told her he was finishing but he didn't want to go to the graduation ceremony. She told him that she wanted to go, so he'd better be there! Tom's mother and Bonnie sat together at graduation. The day had a special meaning for both of them: With their encouragement, Tom had accomplished what he had set out to do.

At twenty-one, Tom still lives with Bonnie and her family and now works full time. She has seen his ability to work hard grow and his relationship with many people blossom, including his mom. "Sometimes people just need space to become the people they can be," Bonnie says. "I did, as a teenager. I argued with my mom a lot. Then a dear friend arranged for me to live with my grandparents, under the pretext that I could go to a better school. Being away gave me the space to appreciate my mother, and we're great friends today. I felt so privileged to be able to pay back what had been given to me. Tom really is a member of our family now, and I love it!"

Like plants, human beings sometimes need a different soil to gain their optimum growth. People like Bonnie, who offer all they have to a child struggling to find himself, are an inspiration for us all. They embody the wisdom of the popular quote, "It takes a whole village to raise a child." When we realize that all children deserve our care, we can create our vision of a new world where all children will receive love and respect for their unique potentials.

Think about children whom you love and want to encourage.

Believe in a New World

If you want the habit of gratitude to grace your life . . .
it is essential that you develop the belief that you are
here on Earth to fulfill some purpose that you can offer
to the world.

M.J. RYAN

Tessie was a six year old in the 1960s. She was one of the African-American girls whose courage psychiatrist Robert Coles tried to understand. Tessie had been among the five children who had helped initiate desegregation in New Orleans. What inner resolve allowed Tessie to walk with the federal marshals through the crowds that were screaming obscenities, yelling that she would die? Tessie held her head high, appearing calm and stoical during the long walk. Searching for the reasons behind her bravery, Coles noted that Tessie drew strength from her handsome, sympathetic grandmother, Martha. This woman had acted in the role of parent, delivering Tessie to the marshals when her mother and father were at work each morning. She talked passionately to her granddaughter about the new world she was helping to create, even though violence threatened all around her.

> You see, my child, you have to help the good Lord
> with His world. He puts us here—and He calls for us
> to help Him out. You belong in that McDonough
> School, and there will be a day when everyone knows
> that, even those poor folks. Lord, I pray for them,
> those poor, poor folks who are shouting their heads

off at you. . . . There's all those people scared out of their minds, and by the time you're ready to leave the McDonough School they'll be calmed down, and they won't be paying you no mind at all, child, and I'll guarantee you, that's how it will be!

During many conversations with Tessie, Coles came to see that she had learned not to look at herself as a victim—a poor black girl, trying to enter a world determined to keep her out—but a child "given the errand of rendering service to a needy population." Her grandmother had convinced Tessie that she was part of God's plan to help give birth to something new in her community and in her country.

Martha had a vision of the world she wanted her children and grandchildren to live in and enjoy. She also had the good fortune to live at a unique time when she could help realize that dream. A few months later, her words to Tessie proved true—people did calm down, and they didn't pay attention to Tessie anymore. Martha could have seen the threats and violence in the sixties South as signs of a coming apocalypse. She could have told her granddaughter that the people who yelled at her were evil and that she should scream back at them. Instead, she told Tessie that they were scared and she should have compassion. She just had to believe that God's plan for the world would prevail.

People like Martha are role models for all of us. We too live at an exceptional hour, and the ways we interpret the events around us will influence what our children believe about the world. The ways we talk about change to our children condition them to view the future as full of hope or foreboding. Our view of this new millennium doesn't have to be created by the sensationalism or fear mongering of the media. It's up to us to see the positive potentials of the age we live in and believe that our children will help create a new world.

The New Troubadours sing a song called "Let New Worlds Grow

from Us." All the world's children need our positive thoughts and prayers. They also need our faith that the way we lead our individual lives matters in making our vision of the world a reality—now while we have the chance.

Write a letter for your child to open in the future about the experiences you hope he has in life. Share the gifts and qualities you believe will help him to do anything he feels inspired to try.

SUGGESTED READING

Doing the Best for Your Child

Apter, Terri. *The Myth of Maturity: What Teenagers Need from Parents to Become Adults*. New York: W. W. Norton, 2000.

Coles, Robert. *The Call of Service: A Witness to Idealism*. New York: Houghton Mifflin, 1993.

Eyre, Richard and Linda. *Teaching Your Children Joy*. New York: Fireside, 1994.

Friedman, Judy S. *Easing the Teasing*. New York: Contemporary Books, 2002.

Ginott, Haim. *Between Parent and Child* (new edition). New York: Three Rivers Press, 2003.

Glasser, Howard and Jennifer Easley. *Transforming the Difficult Child: The Nurtured Heart*. Tucson: Children's Success Foundation, 1998.

Gottmann, John, Joan Declaire, and Daniel P. Goleman, *The Heart of Parenting: How to Raise an Emotionally Intelligent Child*. New York: Simon and Schuster, 1997.

Isaacs, Susan and Wendy Ritchey. *I Think I Can, I Know I Can*. New York: St. Martins Press, 1991.

Kraizer, Sherryll. *The Safe Child Book: A Commonsense Approach to Protecting Children and Teaching Them to Protect Themselves*. New York: Fireside, 1990.

Levine, Mel. *A Mind at a Time*. New York: Simon and Schuster, 2003.

Markova, Dawna. *How Your Child Is Smart: A Life-Changing Approach to Learning*. Berkeley: Conari Press, 1992.

Ricci, Isolina. *Mom's House, Dad's House: Making Two Homes for Your Child*. New York: Fireside, 1997.

Shapiro, Lawrence E. *The Secret Language of Childhood: How to Understand What Your Kids Are Really Saying*. Naperville, IL: Sourcebooks Trade, 2003.

Siegel, Daniel and Mary Hartzell. *Parenting from the Inside Out: How a Deeper Self-Understanding Can Help You Raise Children Who Thrive*. New York: Penguin, 2003.

Simmons, Rachel. *Odd Girl Out: The Hidden Culture of Aggression in Girls*. New York: Harcourt, 2002.

Wolf, Anthony. *The Secret of Parenting: How to Be in Charge of Today's Kids—From Toddlers to Preteens—Without Threats or Punishment*. New York: Farrar, Straus, and Giroux, 2000.

Doing the Best for Yourself

Braner, Lisa Groen. *The Mother's Book of Well-Being*. Boston: Red Wheel/Weiser, 2003

Buckingham, Marcus and Donald Clifton. *Now, Discover Your Strengths*. New York: Free Press, 2001.

Capacchione, Lucia. *The Creative Journal for Parents: A Guide to Unlocking Your Natural Parenting Wisdom*. Boston: Shambhala, 2000.

Carlson, Dr. Richard. *Be Happy No Matter What: Five Principles Your Therapist Never Told You*. Novato, CA: New World Library, 1997.

Faber, Adelle and Elaine Mazlish. *Liberated Parents, Liberated Children*. New York: Avon Books, 1975.

Hay, Louise. *You Can Heal Your Life*. Carlsbad, CA: Hay House, 1999.

Holt, Pat and Grace Keterman. *When You Feel Like Screaming*. Colorado Springs: Shaw, 2000.

Huber, Cheri et al. *Time Out for Themselves: A Compassionate Approach to Parenting*. Mountain View, CA: Compassionworks, 1994.

Lamott, Anne. *Traveling Mercies: Some Thoughts on Faith*. New York: Anchor, 2000.

Lara, Adair. *Hanging Out the Wash: And Other Ways to Find More in Less*. Berkeley: Conari Press, 2002.

Lerner, Harriet. *The Dance of Connection: How to Talk to Someone When You're Mad, Hurt, Scared, Frustrated, Insulted, Betrayed, or Desperate*. New York: Quill, 2002.

Newman, Mildred and Bernard Berkowitz. *How to Be Your Own Best Friend*. New York: Ballantine, 1971.

Ryan, M.J. *Attitudes of Gratitude: How to Give and Receive Joy Every Day of Your Life*. Berkeley: Conari Press, 1999.

Ryan, M.J. *The Power of Patience: How to Slow the Rush and Enjoy More Happiness, Success, and Peace of Mind Every Day*. New York: Broadway Books, 2003.

Seligman, Martin. *Learned Optimism: How to Change Your Mind and Your Life*. New York: Free Press, 1998.

Wilson, Paul. *Instant Calm: Over 100 Easy-to-Use Techniques for Relaxing Mind and Body*. New York: Penguin, 1999.

Zinn, John Kabat. *Full Catastrophe Living: Using the Wisdom of Your Body and Mind to Face Stress, Pain, and Illness*. New York: Bantam Books, 1990.

TOPIC INDEX